PSYCHOSOCIAL HEALTH AND WELL-BEING IN HIGH-LEVEL ATHLETES

The psychological health of competitive athletes is of paramount importance to performance, retention, and well-being in sport, and national governing bodies are increasingly concerned with its promotion. *Psychosocial Health and Well-Being in High-Level Athletes* offers students, researchers, and practicing sport psychologists an accessible and rigorous grounding in the manifestations of psychosocial health in athletes, the threats athletes face to their psychosocial health, and the interventions which can be designed to enhance it.

Seeking to guide future research and expand professional understanding of psychosocial issues in sport, the book is based on a model of cognitive, emotional, social, and spiritual health. It clearly defines these dimensions in a sporting context before discussing pertinent threats—such as career transitions, injuries, and abuse—and interventions, including adversarial growth, life-skill interventions, prevention and organization policy, and mindfulness-based interventions.

Providing an innovative and integrated perspective on psychosocial health and well-being in competitive sport, this book is essential reading for upper-level students taking any clinical sport psychology modules, and for sport psychologists, coaches, and administrators working with competitive athletes.

Nick Galli, Ph.D., CMPC® is an Assistant Professor in the Department of Health, Kinesiology, and Recreation at the University of Utah, USA. Dr. Galli has authored or co-authored more than 20 peer-reviewed articles and book chapters related to psychosocial health in high-level athletes. He was recognized as a distinguished early career scholar by both the Association for Applied Sport Psychology and the American Psychological Association's Society for Sport, Exercise, and Performance Psychology. As a practitioner, Galli serves as the mental performance coach for U.S. speed skating.

PSYCHOSOCIAL HEALTH AND WELL-BEING IN HIGH-LEVEL ATHLETES

Nick Galli

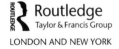
Routledge
Taylor & Francis Group

LONDON AND NEW YORK

First published 2019
by Routledge
2 Park Square, Milton Park, Abingdon, Oxon OX14 4RN

and by Routledge
52 Vanderbilt Avenue, New York, NY 10017

Routledge is an imprint of the Taylor & Francis Group, an informa business

British Library Cataloguing-in-Publication Data
A catalogue record for this book is available from the British Library

Library of Congress Cataloging-in-Publication Data
Names: Galli, Nick, 1979- author.
Title: Psychosocial health and well-being in high-level athletes/Nick Galli.
Description: Abingdon, Oxon; New York, NY: Routledge, 2019. | Includes bibliographical references and index.
Identifiers: LCCN 2018059973 | ISBN 9780815381259 (hardack) | ISBN 9780815381266 (pbk.) | ISBN 9781351210942 (ebook)
Subjects: LCSH: Athletes–Psychology. | Athletes–Mental health. | Sports–Psychological aspects. | Sports–Physiological aspects.
Classification: LCC GV706.4 .G337 2019 | DDC 796.01/9–dc23
LC record available at https://lccn.loc.gov/2018059973

ISBN: 978-0-8153-8125-9 (hbk)
ISBN: 978-0-8153-8126-6 (pbk)
ISBN: 978-1-351-21094-2 (ebk)

Typeset in Bembo
by Deanta Global Publishing Services, Chennai, India

For Julie, Jay, and Bella.

CONTENTS

ILLUSTRATIONS

Figures

Tables

ACKNOWLEDGMENTS

Although the cover shows me (Nick) as sole author, this book is truly the product of interactions and relationships forged over the past 15-plus years. This my opportunity to recognize the individuals who are indirectly responsible for what you are about to read.

First, my primary academic mentors—Dr. Gloria Solomon, Robin Vealey, and Justine Reel. Each of you shaped the knowledge, writing ability, and critical thinking skills that allowed me to craft this book. More importantly, over the years you have become trusted colleagues and friends. Several other teachers and colleagues have been instrumental in my development. Drs. Othello Harris, Mary McDonald, and Thelma Horn taught me to think like a sociologist, which proved unexpectedly valuable for this project! Finally, to my colleagues in Health Promotion and Education at the University of Utah—thanks for taking me in and instilling a health-educator mindset. Their influence is especially apparent in Part III.

A plug for Doris Fortune of Wealth of Words in Salt Lake City, Utah, who worked tirelessly to help get my references in shape prior to submission. Thanks to the crew at the East Millcreek Utah Beans & Brews for keeping me caffeine-fueled as I typed day in and day out at your establishment. Last, but not least, thanks to the athletes and researchers whose efforts provided the source material for this project. Without you, there is no book.

PART I

Foundations of psychosocial health

Before focusing on specific threats to athletes' psychosocial health, or proposing ideas for the prevention and management of psychosocial health issues, it is first necessary to provide a conceptual foundation and establish a common language from which to discuss these issues. Although in practice it is nearly impossible to consider the different domains of health and well-being in isolation, for didactic purposes it is beneficial to consider them separately. In *Chapter 1*, I define key terms, offer an overview of research on well-being in sport, and highlight the importance of considering the psychosocial aspects of health for both athletic performance and global well-being.

In *Chapter 2*, I introduce the cognitive and emotional domains of psychosocial health. Due to its implications for skill-learning and within-competition decision-making, the cognitive domain of psychosocial health is especially linked to sport performance. Beyond performance, sport can serve both as an enhancer and debilitator of important cognitive functions. Emotional health (often referred to as mental health) has received increased attention from elite sport organizations, due in part to several high-profile athletes speaking out about their conditions. Scholarly research on emotional health in athletes has also increased, and I share important findings relative to the prevalence of emotional health issues in sport, as well as the conditions under which sport may serve as a risk or protective factor for such issues.

Finally, *Chapter 3* highlights the relevance of social and spiritual health for high-level athletes. Social health has most often been examined through the lens of Keyes' (1998) theory of social well-being, which is one component of psychological well-being. In addition to reviewing two studies of social well-being in athletes, I synthesize the literature related to social support. I conclude the chapter with an introduction to spiritual health, which has most often been studied in athletes as spirituality or religiousness. Specifically, I discuss research suggesting competitive sport as an ideal site for the expression and realization of spiritual health, as well as the link between spiritual health and the emotional and social dimensions of psychosocial health.

1

THE RELEVANCE OF PSYCHOSOCIAL HEALTH FOR HIGH-LEVEL ATHLETES

Garrett is a professional basketball player who has recently been traded to a new team. As part of the trade, his new team requires him to undergo a physical exam to ensure that he is healthy to train and compete. The exam is comprehensive, and includes questions on Garrett's medical history (e.g., past injuries), as well as biometric assessments such as heart rate, blood pressure, vision, and a general evaluation of posture, range of motion, and muscle strength. The physician gives Garrett a clean bill of health, and the trade is finalized. Things are going well until about mid-season, when Garrett begins arriving late to practice, missing team meetings, and performing below his usual standard. Upon being confronted by his coach and teammates, Garrett admits to having struggled on-and-off with his emotions for several years and agrees to get help from a mental health professional. After his in-take session with the therapist, Garrett is diagnosed with major depressive disorder, and begins a program of medication combined with regular psychotherapy. The front-office staff decides that future physical exams should go beyond the physical aspects of athletes' health.

High-performing athletes are revered for their remarkable feats of strength, speed, and endurance. Elite-level endurance athletes such as cross-country skiers can use almost twice the amount of oxygen as a typically trained adult (Hutchinson, 2014), and weightlifters who compete at the Olympics routinely lift two to three times their body weight from the floor to above their heads (Anon., 2012). Athletes in team sports possess an uncanny ability to quickly assess the situation and react to constantly changing circumstances, all while coordinating their actions with those of their teammates. Athletes who have achieved such impressive feats on the playing field are often called upon to be role models of healthy living (Lisanti, 2017). Paradoxically, these same high-performing athletes often struggle with a variety of health issues, including life-altering injuries, coach abuse, drug and alcohol dependence, and disordered eating behaviors (Safai, Fraser-Thomas, & Baker, 2015). Unfortunately, as seen in the hypothetical case of Garrett, such issues are often taken for granted by sport organizations.

The varied meanings of health

Before engaging in a critical discussion of athlete health, it is first necessary to discuss both how the term is commonly used in sport, as well as define how it will be used in this text. To illustrate the typical view of health in sport, imagine the head coach of a high-level team addressing the media prior to an important game or match. As reporters pepper her with questions, the subject of certain team members' health naturally arises. Regardless of her response, the implied context is the physical status of the athlete in question. An expected answer might be "Player X has been cleared by the team doctor to play in today's game," or "Player Y has a stomach virus and will be out of action tonight." Such answers reveal important assumptions about the nature of health. First, it seems clear that the coach has adopted a medical-model view, in which health is viewed as the mere absence of disease or injury (Laing, 1971). Second, it is exceedingly rare for a coach, athlete, or team official to address athlete health from a holistic perspective; instead, they tend to reduce the issue to one of physical illness or injury. That is, even if an athlete was struggling with a psychosocial health concern such as a bout of depression that put his ability to play in jeopardy, such issues are usually either not discussed, or not immediately considered as fitting under the purview of athlete health.

In this text I will adopt the World Health Organization's more versatile definition of health as "a state of complete physical, mental and social well-being and not merely the absence of disease or infirmity" (WHO, 1946). Although some health concerns of athletes, such as injury, have clear physical implications, rarely are the antecedents and consequences of such concerns *purely* physical. Depending on the severity of the injury, athletes can expect to experience a variety of cognitive, emotional, social, and even spiritual challenges in the process of recovery (Clement, Arvinen-Barrow, & Fetty, 2015). Substance dependence, although certainly a physical threat to athletes, is also often the result of social pressure to perform, and can in turn have profound psychological effects (Whitaker, Long, Petróczi, & Backhouse, 2013). Thus, a more complete approach to athlete health extends beyond the physical to include the cognitive (i.e., thinking), emotional (i.e., feeling), social (i.e., relating with others), and spiritual (i.e., connection with something greater than oneself) dimensions (Donatelle, 2015). For example, a collegiate volleyball player who recently transferred to a different university will ideally learn the strategy of her new team at an appropriate rate (i.e., cognitive health), effectively cope with the stress of transition (i.e., emotional health), form new productive relationships on and off the court (i.e., social health), and feel a sense of purpose and fulfillment as it relates to her academic and athletic career (i.e., spiritual health).

Taken together, these four dimensions of psychosocial health can be viewed as an indicator of athletes' *well-being,* or "diverse and interconnected physical, mental, and social factors extending beyond traditional definitions of health" (Naci & Ioannidis, 2015, p. 121). As depicted in Figure 1.1, athletes' psychosocial health and well-being are under constant bombardment from threats such as injury and transition (see Chapters 4–8). With careful planning, negative health concerns can be prevented (see Chapters 9–10). However, even the best prevention cannot eliminate all health concerns, and later-stage prevention and treatment are often warranted (see Chapter 11). Finally, for some athletes, the experience of health concerns and/or the process of treatment may be an opportunity for displays of resilience or the realization of personal growth (see Chapter 12).

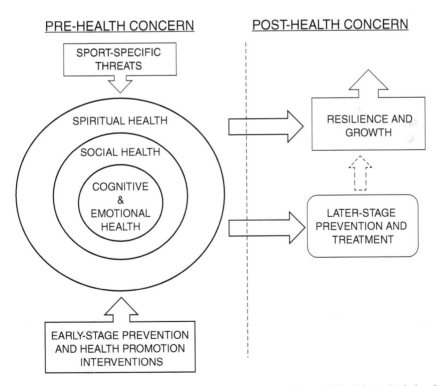

FIGURE 1.1 A conceptual model for understanding psychosocial health in high-level athletes

Well-being

Because the concept of well-being is, in and of itself, of interest to sport research-ers, it warrants specific consideration. Numerous scholars have offered models of well-being in the general population, which usually involve some combina-tion of social and emotional dimensions. For example, in his tripartite model of subjective well-being, Diener (1984) posited that degree of positive and negative affect (i.e., affective balance) and life satisfaction determine individuals' well-being. Ryff's (1989) six-factor model of psychological well-being emphasizes the factors of self-acceptance, personal growth, life purpose, environmental mastery, autonomy, and positive relations with others as forming the foundation of well-being. Central to current conceptions of well-being is the distinction between *hedonic* well-being (i.e., subjective well-being), or individuals' subjective experi-ences of happiness, and *eudaimonic* well-being (i.e., psychological well-being), or the extent to which individuals pursue meaningful goals leading to personal fulfillment. A further component of psychological well-being (PWB) is *social well-being,* or individuals' perception of the extent to which their social life is flourishing (Keyes, 1998). Social well-being is further divided into five com-ponents: (a) social acceptance, (b) social actualization, (c) social contribution, (d) social coherence, and (e) social integration. Each of these five components is discussed in Chapter 3.

It should be noted that Ryff and Diener's conceptions of well-being represent a decidedly Westernized (i.e., individualistic) view of the construct, and some have questioned whether such a view accurately represents the experiences of individuals from more Eastern (i.e., collectivistic) cultures found in Asian and Middle Eastern countries (Lu & Gilmour, 2004; Suhail & Chaudhry, 2004). Eastern versus Western differences in the experience of subjective well-being (SWB) have been of interest to researchers who contend that happiness is cul-ture-dependent. For example, Lu and Gilmour (2004) compared Chinese and American university students' responses to the question "What is happiness?" They found that, as opposed to American students, who associated happiness with certain mental and emotional states, personal achievement, and autonomy, Chinese students tended to focus more on maintaining a sense of balance, or homeostasis, between themselves and their environment. Thus, although in this text I will primarily present views of health and well-being reflective of Western views (as nearly all of the research has been conducted with North American and European populations), readers should be aware that what counts as *healthy* and *well* is highly dependent on cultural norms and values.

When applying the Western view of well-being to athletes, from a hedonic perspective, an athlete may experience well-being in the form of happiness and pride in setting a new personal record time. This same athlete may also experi-ence eudaimonic well-being due to training and competing in accordance with their personal values of being a strong role model, being coachable, and compet-ing with integrity (see Table 1.1).

TABLE 1.1 Characteristics of hedonic and eudaimonic aspects of well-being for athletes

	Hedonic Well-Being	Eudaimonic Well-Being
Frame of reference	Subjective (e.g., "I feel happy with my performance.")	Objective (e.g., "I am mentally stronger due to my sport injury.")
Meaning	Personal happiness	Cultivation of personal strengths; contribution to greater society
Common terms	"Happiness," "Pleasure," "Enjoyment"	"Fulfillment," "Personal growth," "Purpose"

In her comprehensive treatment of well-being research conducted in sport through 2010, Lundqvist (2011) noted an inconsistency in how researchers chose to operationalize well-being. From a hedonic perspective, the construct has been operationalized as the self-reported presence or absence of positive and negative emotions as measured by inventories such as the Positive and Negative Affect Scale (PANAS; Watson, Clark, & Tellegen, 1988), and/or as measured by psychological traits and states such as body satisfaction and self-esteem (e.g., Martin DiBartolo & Shaffer, 2002; Reinboth & Duda, 2004). Even among researchers who did clearly state their orientation toward well-being (i.e., subjective vs. psychological), Lundqvist (2011) noted a failure to use assessments which align with the stated orientation. Inspection of the literature on well-being in sport published since Lundqvist's review shows a general improvement in both the specification of researchers' orientation to well-being and the alignment of this orientation to assessment (e.g., Ferguson, Kowalski, Mack, & Sabiston, 2014; Jeon, Lee, & Kwon, 2016; Lundqvist & Raglin, 2015). For example, in their study of well-being in injured athletes, Lu and Hsu (2013) clearly articulated their interest in subjective well-being, and chose measurements that fit with this approach—the Trait Hope Scale and the Chinese version of the PANAS.

In response to the lack of conceptual clarity within research on well-being in sport, Lundqvist (2011) proposed an athlete-specific model of well-being. The model is informed both by conceptualizations of well-being in general, and extant research on well-being in sport. As seen in Figure 1.2, the model accounts for global and sport-specific well-being, as well as hedonic and eudaimonic dimensions of well-being. The resulting model allows for a multi-dimensional view of well-being in sport, in which athlete well-being can be understood across six domains: (a) global subjective well-being (i.e., life satisfaction), (b) sport subjective well-being (i.e., sport satisfaction), (c) global psychological well-being (i.e., life purpose), (d) sport psychological well-being (i.e., purpose in sport), (e) global social well-being (i.e., general social acceptance), and (f) sport social well-being (i.e., social acceptance in sport).

Using the model as a guide, Lundqvist and Sandin (2014) interviewed ten elite orienteers to explore factors characterizing the different forms of well-being. Hedonic indicators of well-being such as life satisfaction and sport enjoyment

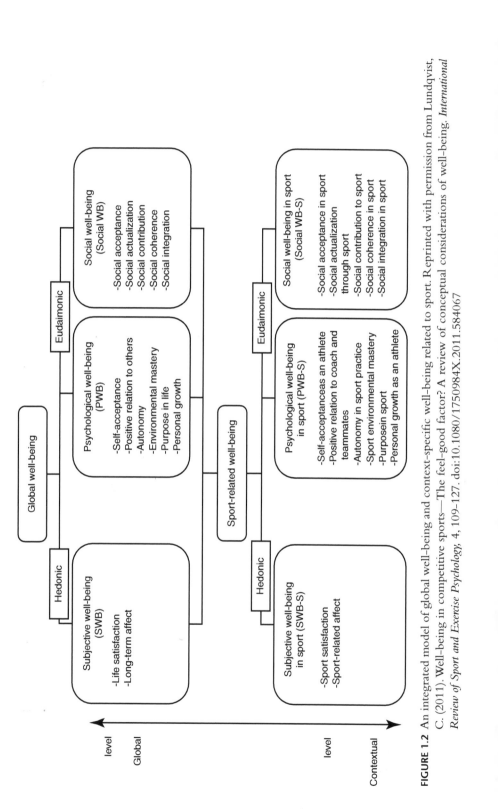

FIGURE 1.2 An integrated model of global well-being and context-specific well-being related to sport. Reprinted with permission from Lundqvist, C. (2011). Well-being in competitive sports—The feel-good factor? A review of conceptual considerations of well-being. *International Review of Sport and Exercise Psychology*, 4, 109–127. doi:10.1080/1750984X.2011.584067

interacted with eudaimonic indicators such as autonomy and personal growth to produce orienteers' well-being experience. Further, orienteers' global, non-sport specific well-being at a given point in time served as the foundation for their sport well-being. This finding highlights the importance of adopting a holistic approach to athletes' health and well-being emphasizing both sport and non-sport aspects.

Sport as an enhancer or debilitator of optimal psychosocial health and well-being

Although much has been written about the role of sport in shaping desirable (or undesirable) psychosocial qualities in youth (e.g., Ferris, Ettekal, Agans, & Burkhard, 2015), the psychosocial health and well-being of adult athletes competing at a high-level have been mostly ignored. Importantly, this includes a focus on the potential for competitive sport to *undermine* psychosocial health. As Safai, Fraser-Thomas, and Baker (2015) articulated about the documentary *Road to the Olympics* in their text *Health and Elite Sport*:

> As social scientists who study health and sport, we were struck by the paradox of experiences that made up these Olympians' journeys. We recognized their incredible physical capabilities of fitness, strength, and skill, their psychological motivation, determination and focus, coupled with their widespread appeal as models of health, work ethic, sportspersonship and character. But we were also struck by the notable and consistent attention paid to pain and injury as part of each athlete's personal story.
>
> *(p. 1)*

Indeed, such pain often extends to include the cognitive and emotional domains of athlete health, such as when gymnasts develop distorted views about the size and shape of their bodies (Neves, Meireles, de Carvalho, Schubring, Barker-Ruchti, Caputo Ferreira, 2017), American football players choose to withhold symptoms of head trauma (Kuhn, Zuckerman, Yengo-Kahn, Kerr, Totten, Rubel, Sills, & Solomon, 2017), and elite athletes struggle with the transition from competition to a "normal" life (Cosh, Crabb, & Tully, 2015). As discussed further in Chapter 5, when the sport culture is designed with performance and winning as the primary value, athletes are more likely to push themselves in unhealthy ways, and are often celebrated for their efforts in doing so (Hughes & Coakley, 1991). The pressure on coaches to deliver championships can exacerbate the situation, as they may at best be complicit in athletes' unhealthy pursuit of glory, and at worst resort to physical and emotional abuse in the name of performance (Stirling & Kerr, 2015). As prominent governing bodies of sport such as the National Collegiate Athletics Association (NCAA) and the English Institute of Sport (EIS) begin to prioritize athlete well-being independent of performance, sport researchers and professionals need a comprehensive resource in this area.

In this book I synthesize current research related to psychosocial health in high-level athletes, and offer suggestions for future research and practice related to the psychosocial health and well-being of high-level athletes. For the purpose of this text, I define *high-level* sport participants as those who devote significant time and resources to training and competition, and who compete regularly at the regional, national, international, or professional level. Figure 1.1 is a schematic representation of this text. The concentric circles depict each of the four dimensions of psychosocial health, from those elements most central to the athlete to those elements most external (Chapters 2–3). The boxed arrow pointing downward from above the circles represents common threats to athletes' psychosocial health, including organizational stress, psychological pressure to perform, abuse, injury, and transition. At the core of threats to the psychosocial health of athletes is the aforementioned "win-at-all-costs" culture of high-level collegiate, international, and professional sport. The boxed arrow pointing upward from below the circles represents primary, secondary, and tertiary approaches used to prevent adverse psychosocial outcomes in high-level athletes (Chapters 9–11). Finally, the bent upward pointing arrow to the right of the circles illustrates the potential for resilience and psychosocial growth in athletes due to the experience of threats to psychosocial health (Chapter 12).

References

Anon. (2012, July 29). *North Korean Olympian lifts 3 times his weight. CBS News.* Retrieved from https://www.cbsnews.com/news/north-korean-olympian-lifts-3-times-his-weight/

Clement, D., Arvinen-Barrow, M., & Fetty, T. (2015). Psychosocial responses during different phases of sport-injury rehabilitation: A qualitative study. *Journal of Athletic Training, 50*(1), 95–104. doi:10.4085/1062-6050-49.3.52

Cosh, S., Crabb, S., & Tully, P. J. (2015). A champion out of the pool? A discursive exploration of two Australian Olympic swimmers' transition from elite sport to retirement. *Psychology of Sport and Exercise, 19,* 33e41. Retrieved from http://www.pasap.eu/wp-content/uploads/2015/04/Australians-Swimmers-2015.pdf

DiBartolo, D. M., & Shaffer, C. (2002). A comparison of female college athletes and nonathletes: Eating disorder symptomatology and psychological well-being. *Journal of Sport & Exercise Psychology, 24.* doi:10.1123/jsep.24.1.33

Diener, E. (1984). Subjective well-being. *Psychological Bulletin, 95*(3), 542–575.

Donatelle, R. J. (2015). *Health: The basics* (11th ed.). Pearson eText. Retrieved from https://www.pearson.com/us/higher-education/product/Donatelle-Health-The-Basics-11th-Edition/9780321910424.html?tab=resources

Ferguson, L. J., Kowalski, K. C., Mack, D. E., & Sabiston, C. M. (2014). Exploring self-compassion and eudaimonic well-being in young women athletes. *Journal of Sport & Exercise Psychology, 36,* 203–216. doi:10.1123/jsep.2013-0096

Ferris, K. A., Ettekal, A. V., Agans, J. P., & Burkhard, B. M. (2015). Character development through youth sport: High school coaches' perspectives about a character-based education program. *Journal of Youth Development, 10*(3), 127–140. doi:10.5195/jyd.2015.13

Hughes, R., & Coakley, J. (1991). Positive deviance among athletes: The implications of overconformity to the sport ethic. *Sociology of Sport Journal, 8,* 307–325.

Hutchinson, A. (2014). Who has the greatest VO2max of them all? *Runner's World*. Retrieved from https://www.runnersworld.com/training/a20832549/who-has-the-greatest-vo2max-of-them-all/

Jeon, H., Lee, K., & Kwon, S. (2016). Investigation of the structural relationships between social support, self-compassion, and subjective well-being in Korean elite student athletes. *Psychological Reports, 119*(1), 39–54. doi:10.1177/0033294116658226

Kerr, G. A., & Stirling, A. E. (2015). Professionalization of coaches to reduce emotionally harmful coaching practices: Lessons learned from the education sector. *International Journal of Coaching Science, 9*(1), 21–36.

Keyes, C. L. M. (1998). Social well-being. *Social Psychology Quarterly, 61*(2), 121. doi:10.2307/2787065

Kuhn, A. W., Zuckerman, S. L., Yengo-Kahn, A. M., Kerr, Z. Y., Totten, D. J., Rubel, K. E., … Solomon, G. S. (2017). Factors associated with playing through a sport-related concussion. *Neurosurgery, 64*(Suppl. 1), 211–216. doi:10.1093/neuros/nyx294

Laing, R. D. (1971). *The politics of the family and other essays.* New York, NY: Pantheon Books.

Lisanti, J. (2017). Body count. *Sports Illustrated, 127*(9), 40–45.

Lu, L., & Gilmour, R. (2004). Culture and conceptions of happiness: Individual oriented and social oriented SWB. *Journal of Happiness Studies, 5*(3), 269–291. doi:10.1007/s10902-004-8789-5

Lu, F. J.-H., & Hsu, Y. (2013). Injured athletes' rehabilitation beliefs and subjective well-being: The contribution of hope and social support. *Journal of Athletic Training, 48*(1), 92–98. doi:10.4085/1062-6050-48.1.03

Lundqvist, C. (2011). Well-being in competitive sports—The feel-good factor? A review of conceptual considerations of well-being. *International Review of Sport and Exercise Psychology, 4*(2), 109–127. doi:10.1080/1750984X.2011.584067

Lundqvist, C., & Raglin, J. S. (2015). The relationship of basic need satisfaction, motivational climate and personality to well-being and stress patterns among elite athletes: An explorative study. *Motivation and Emotion, 39*(2), 237–246. doi:10.1007/s11031-014-9444-z

Lundqvist, C., & Sandin, F. (2014). Well-being in elite sport: Dimensions of hedonic and eudaimonic well-being among elite orienteers. *Sport Psychologist, 28*(3), 245–254. doi:10.1123/tsp.2013-0024

Naci, H., & Ioannidis, J. P. A. (2015). Evaluation of wellness determinants and interventions by citizen scientists. *JAMA, 314*(2), 121–122. doi:10.1001/jama.2015.6160

Neves, C. M., Meireles, J. F. F., de Carvalho, P. H. B., Schubring, A., Barker-Ruchti, N., & Caputo Ferreira, M. E. (2017). Body dissatisfaction in women's artistic gymnastics: A longitudinal study of psychosocial indicators. *Journal of Sports Sciences, 35*(17), 1745–1751. doi:10.1080/02640414.2016.1235794

Reinboth, M., & Duda, J. L. (2004). The motivational climate, perceived ability, and athletes' psychological and physical well-being. *The Sport Psychologist, 18*(3), 237–251. doi:10.1123/tsp.18.3.237

Ryff, C. D. (1989). Happiness is everything, or is it? Explorations on the meaning of psychological well-being. *Journal of Personality and Social Psychology, 57*, 1069–1081. doi:10.1037/0022-3514.57.6.1069

Suhail, K., & Chaudhry, H. R. (2004). Predictors of subjective well-being in an eastern Muslim culture. *Journal of Social and Clinical Psychology, 23*(3), 359–376. doi:10.1521/jscp.23.3.359.35451

Safai, P., Fraser-Thomas, J., & Baker, J. (2015). Sport and health of the high performance athlete: An introduction to the text. In J. Baker, P. Safai, & J. Fraser-Thomas

(Eds.), *Health and elite sport: Is high performance sport a healthy pursuit?* New York, NY: Routledge, Taylor & Francis Group.

Stirling, A., & Kerr, G. (2015). Safeguarding athletes from emotional abuse. In M. Lang, & M. Harthill (Eds.), *Safeguarding, Child Protection and Abuse in Sport: International Perspectives in Research*, Policy and Practice (pp.143–152), London: Routledge Press.

Watson, D., Clark, L. A., & Tellegen, A. (1988). Development and validation of brief measures of positive and negative affect: The PANAS Scales. *Journal of Personality and Social Psychology, 54*(6), 1063–1070. Retrieved from http://www.cnbc.pt/jpmatos/28. Watson.pdf

Whitaker, L., Long, J., Petróczi, A., & Backhouse, S. (2013). Using the prototype willingness model to predict doping in sport. *Scandinavian Journal of Medicine and Science in Sports, 24.* doi:10.1111/sms.12148

2

COGNITIVE AND EMOTIONAL HEALTH

Shayla is a 19-year-old collegiate water polo goalie. As with most of her teammates, Shayla displays excellence both in terms of her cognitive skills (e.g., processing speed, executive functioning), and emotional stability (e.g., emotional intelligence, subjective and objective well-being). During a scrimmage during practice one day, a teammate inadvertently hits Shayla in the side of her head with an elbow. Upon being assessed by the team's athletic trainer, it is determined that Shayla has sustained a concussion. Over the weeks to come Shayla experiences persistent headaches, nausea, and uncommon sensory overload while in public places. Follow-up assessments revealed decrements in Shayla's processing speed and reaction time as compared to pre-concussion. Perhaps even more disturbing were the changes to her mood, as she often found herself crying for seemingly no reason.

Shayla's story depicts the paradox of high-level sport, in which athletes' cognitive and emotional health can be at once bolstered and degraded due to the demands of training and competition. As illustrated in Figure 1.1, psychosocial health can be viewed as concentric, with the elements more internal to the athlete closer to the center. This chapter includes a focus on the two inner-most elements of psychosocial health—cognitive and emotional.

Cognitive health

Cognition refers broadly to internal processes involved in learning, attention, memory, problem-solving, and decision-making (Gerrig, 2012). Functions contributing to cognitive health, including sensorimotor (e.g., gross and fine motor skills), executive functioning (e.g., planning, organizing, and evaluating), intellect (e.g., problem-solving), attention (e.g., ability to focus on a task), language (e.g., ability to comprehend and communicate effectively), emotions (e.g., subjective feelings), memory (e.g., ability to store and retrieve information), and visual-spatial (e.g., ability to make sense of visual world). Individuals who are cognitively healthy think clearly, learn at an appropriate rate, and adopt effective decision-making strategies (National Institute of Neurological Disorders and Stroke [NINDS], National Institute of Mental Health [NIMH], & National Institute of Aging [NIA], 2001). Although some of the cognitive functions are particularly relevant to athletic performance (e.g., visual-spatial, sensorimotor), all are important for athletes' activities of daily living.

Of all the domains of psychosocial health, cognitive health is perhaps the one most closely linked to on-field athletic performance. For example, a golfer must have the ability to comprehend and implement their coach's technical swing instructions during a competitive round. The very best baseball and softball players are adept at successfully modifying their game plan for particular hitters and pitchers. And elite short-track speedskaters make split-second decisions about whether to pass an opponent while traveling at speeds up to 30 miles per hour. Thus, despite stereotypes perpetuating the myth of the "dumb jock," (Simons, Bosworth, Fujita, & Jensen, 2007), exceptional athletes are some of the most cognitively healthy individuals in the world.

Athletes' cognitive health has been examined both in terms of within-sport expertise (i.e., expert performance approach), and in terms of the transfer of such expertise outside the sport domain (i.e., cognitive component skill approach). Regarding the former, athletes' advanced visual tracking, pattern recall, and decision-making is sport-specific, and develops over the course of thousands of hours/repetitions on tasks specific to a given sport (Williams & Ericsson, 2005). Perhaps more relevant for the overall psychosocial health of athletes is the cognitive component skill approach, as it suggests a positive transfer of important skills such as executive functioning and visual tracking from the playing field to everyday life.

In one study by Faubert (2013), non-athlete university students, professional and elite amateur athletes were each tested on their ability to learn a context-neutral sphere tracking and identification task over the course of fifteen 8-minute sessions. The results showed that, as compared to elite amateurs and non-athletes, professional athletes learned the task at a much quicker rate. Similarly, the amateurs' rate of learning was superior to that of non-athletes. In a study by Chaddock, Neider, Voss, Gaspar, and Kramer (2011), collegiate athletes and non-athletes were compared on their ability to successfully complete a virtual-reality task requiring them to safely walk across a virtual street while simultaneously talking on a cell phone or listening to music. Interestingly, despite moving at the same speed, athletes were successful in crossing the street significantly more often than non-athletes. The authors concluded that athletes possessed superior processing speed which allowed them to more expertly multitask than non-athletes. Thus, it seems that even when the context is neutral, cognitive abilities differ as a function of sport participation and competitive level. These findings support the role of sport in enhancing general cognitive abilities outside of the competitive context.

Cognitive health and Masters athletes

The cognitive health domain is particularly germane to the experience of individuals who compete in Masters athletics, defined by World Masters Athletics (WMA) as individuals aged 35 and above. Because declines in memory, reasoning, and comprehension can occur in individuals as young as 45 (Singh-Manoux, Kivimaki, Glymour, Elbaz, Berr, Ebmeier, Ferrie, & Dugravot, 2012), and because physical activity may attenuate such declines (Garcia-Hermoso, Ramírez-Vélez, Celis-Morales, Olloquequi, & Izquierdo, 2018), older adults who participate in competitive sport may be somewhat protected from age-related degenerative changes in cognitive health.

Research supports the contention that sport participation has a positive effect on cognitive health. In one study, the researchers used magnetic resonance imaging (MRI) to compare the brain tissue concentration between female Masters athletes (M = 72.4 years) and an age- and education-matched group of sedentary women (M = 74.6 years). The findings revealed that the athlete group had significantly higher concentrations of gray and white matter than the sedentary group in areas of the brain responsible for visuospatial function, working memory, and motor control (Tseng, Uh, Rossetti, Cullum, Diaz-Arrastia, Levine, Lu, & Zhang, 2013). Unfortunately, the study by Tseng et al. is the only one to date linking sport participation with cognitive health benefits in Masters athletes. Many questions remain—including whether there are differential cognitive benefits of competing in endurance activities such as running versus team sports such as basketball, and whether early sport participation plays a role in later cognitive status. Researchers will need to employ longitudinal studies including both brain-imaging procedures and cognitive testing to fully understand the relationship between sport participation and cognitive health.

Assessment of cognitive health and function in athletes

Because athletes' cognitive abilities are believed to contribute to performance, for years elite and professional sport teams have adopted cognitive-testing procedures to identify athletes who are best able to "think on their feet" and display a high "game IQ." However, these tests are often criticized for not generalizing well to specific sport contexts. For example, quarterback Dan Marino scored 15 out of 50 (a below-average score) on the Wonderlic Personnel Test (Wonderlic & Hovland, 1939), and went on to become one of the greatest quarterbacks in National Football League history. Furthermore, a study by Lyons, Hoffman, and Michel (2009) found no relationship between Wonderlic scores and future games started and performance in 762 NFL players. A more recent attempt to measure athlete intelligence was by Scott Goldman, who developed the Athlete Intelligence Quotient (AIQ) as a way to measure the cognitive qualities most closely associated with sport performance (Athletic Intelligence Measures, 2018). Based on the Cattell-Horn-Carroll Theory of Intelligence (Carroll, 2003), the AIQ conceptualizes athlete intelligence as multidimensional, and allows for the assessment of those cognitive abilities most relevant for performance, including memory, reaction time, visual processing, and processing speed. Rather than rely solely on written questions, the AIQ consists of hands-on problem-solving tasks that athletes complete on a computerized tablet. The AIQ has shown some promise for predicting baseball hitting and pitching performance (Athletic Intelligence Measures, 2017), and it will be interesting to see whether it begins to replace the Wonderlic as the cognitive test of choice among talent evaluators.

Critical thinking

One important aspect of cognitive health not typically assessed by talent evaluators is *critical thinking*, or "the ability to assess claims based on well-supported reasoning … [and] resist claims that have no supporting evidence (Wade & Tavris, 1998, p. 4–5)." Not only is critical thinking important for optimal on-field decision-making (e.g., a soccer forward taking a calculated risk based on the situation rather than the conventional approach when trying to score), but off the field as well (e.g., rejecting long-held but harmful "traditions" such as hazing). When athletes are part of a system in which they are expected to act as "subordinates" and faithful rule-followers to coaches and administrators, critical thinking may suffer (McBride & Reed, 1998). Such unquestioned obedience to authority and inability to "think outside the box" may have roots in organized elite youth sport, where children learn rigid rules and strategies without the opportunity for creative self-expression or decision-making responsibility (Coakley, 1992; Ginsburg, 2007). Further research is necessary to understand the conditions under which critical thinking is hindered or facilitated by sport.

Concussions

Beyond the potential undermining of critical thinking skills, sports involving a high degree of physical contact can prove problematic for athletes' cognitive health. In particular, popular sports such as American football pose a high risk for *concussions*, which are defined by the Centers for Disease Control as a "traumatic brain injury caused by a bump, blow, or jolt to the head … that causes the head and brain to move rapidly back and forth." Athletes who experience a concussion, estimated at between 1.6 and 3.8 million sport participants annually (Langlois, Rutland-Brown, & Wald, 2006), may experience short- and long-term deficits in memory, processing, and attention (Moore, Hillman, & Broglio, 2014). The issue of concussions in sport has recently been brought to light by several high-profile athletes such as Sidney Crosby of the National Hockey League, whose own concussions between 2011 and 2017 not only resulted in missed playing time, but persistent headaches caused by everyday activities such as watching television or driving (Pittsburgh's Action News 4, 2017). The issue of concussions is further compounded by the unquestioning acceptance of the norms of high-level sport, as athletes may attempt to conceal symptoms and/or choose to "fight through" in order to retain their spot on the team, or because they don't believe that their symptoms are severe enough to warrant sitting out (Beidler, Bretzin, Hancock, & Covassin, 2017; Delaney, Lamfookon, Bloom, Al-Kashmiri, & Correa, 2015). The wide-ranging psychosocial health implications of concussions for athletes are discussed further in Chapter 7.

Conclusion

In sum, the cognitive domain of health is essential for the optimal functioning and performance of high-level athletes both on and off the playing field. Although the controlling structure of competitive sport may stifle athletes' critical thinking, top athletes tend to be superior to non-athletes on most cognitive abilities, and research suggests that these abilities can generalize to non-sport activities. For Masters level athletes, competitive sport participation appears to offer protection from age-related declines in cognitive function. Concussions are a serious threat to athletes' cognitive health, and are discussed further in Chapter 7.

Emotional health

Although the World Health Organization (2014) defines *mental health* as a state in which individuals realize their own potential, effectively cope with the normal stresses of life, work productively, and contribute to their community, it is also frequently used interchangeably with the term mental *illness* (beyondblue, n.d.; Canadian Mental Health Association, 2015). Because of the inconsistent use of the term mental health, and because emotions are closely linked to mental health, I instead use the term *emotional health* in reference to the aforementioned definition. As noted by the National Institutes of Health (NIH, 2001), it is impossible to consider cognitive and mental/emotional health separately, as emotions are intricately tied to cognitive processes. However, for the purposes of clarity and organization, in this chapter I address them separately.

Primary emotional health issues for adults

Although a comprehensive description of all emotional health issues is beyond the scope of this text, I will briefly describe the issues that are of primary concern for both athletes and the general population. *Anxiety* is a negative emotion involving feelings of tension, worry, and physiological changes. According to the Harvard

Medical School's National Comorbidity Study (NCS; 2017), 19.2% of adults in the United States (U.S.) were diagnosed with some form of anxiety disorder between 2001 and 2003, and an estimated 31.3% of U.S. adults were diagnosed at some point in their lives. A common emotional health concern often co-existing with anxiety is *depression,* which "refers to a mood disorder that causes a persistent feeling of sadness and loss of interest" (Mayo Clinic, 2018). According to Substance Abuse and Mental Health Services Administration (Substance Abuse and Mental Health Services Administration [SAMHSA], 2015), over 16 million (6.7%) of U.S. adults experienced a depressive episode in 2015.

The experience of clinical anxiety and/or depression can co-occur with, or serve as a trigger to, pathological behaviors such as substance abuse and disordered eating. SAMHSA (2015) defines *substance abuse* as "the recurrent use of alcohol and/or drugs causing clinically and functionally significant impairment, such as health problems, disability, and failure to meet major responsibilities at work, school, or home." For example, in 2014 about 17 million individuals in the U.S. had an alcohol use disorder, and about 1.9 million people had an opioid abuse disorder (SAMHSA, 2015). Eating disorders, characterized by the Diagnostic and Statistical Manual of Mental Disorders-5 as a range of abnormal eating habits that negatively affect a person's physical or mental health (American Psychiatric Association [APA], 2013), represent another emotional health threat. For women, the lifetime prevalence of anorexia nervosa (AN) is between 0.9 and 2%, the lifetime prevalence of bulimia nervosa (BN) is between 1.1 and 4.6%, and the lifetime prevalence of binge eating disorder (BED) is between 0.2 and 3.5% (Stice & Bohon, 2013). For men, the lifetime prevalence of AN is between 0.1 and 0.3%, the lifetime prevalence of BN is between 0.1 and 0.5%, and the lifetime prevalence of BED is between 0.9 and 2%. AN is not only the deadliest of all eating disorders, but of all emotional health issues. In a 2011 meta-analysis, Arcelus, Mitchell, Wales, and Nielsen calculated the weighted mortality rate of AN as 5.1 per 1000 people-years, which is almost five times the rate of BN. An additional proportion of individuals will experience subclinical manifestations of eating disorders, which can also have debilitative health outcomes. For example, up to 5.4% of adolescent women will develop subclinical BN in their lives (Stice & Bohon, 2013). Although the statistics revealed in this section are not athletes, athletes are a unique population, who, depending on the nature of their experience, may be more or less protected from such issues. I now shift to a focus on the study of emotional health in athletes.

Early research on emotional health in athletes

Upon recognition as an academic sub-discipline in the 1960s and 1970s, much of the early U.S. research in sport psychology focused on the personality traits of athletes versus non-athletes (e.g., Slusher, 1964), or less successful versus more successful athletes (e.g., Schurr, Ashley, & Joy, 1977). The most influential model to arise from this period was William Morgan's (1979) Mental Health Model.

A clinician by training, Morgan was one of the first psychologists in the U.S. to regularly administer tests of emotional health such as the Minnesota Multiphasic Personality Inventory (MMPI), the Eysenck Personality Inventory, and the State-Trait Anxiety Inventory (STAI) to collegiate and elite athletes (Morgan, 1979).

However, Morgan's most notable contribution to the study of emotional health in high-level athletes involved the use of the Profile of Mood States (POMS; McNair, Droppleman, & Lorr, 1971), a 65-item instrument designed to measure six dimensions of mood: (a) Tension or Anxiety, (b) Anger or Hostility, (c) Vigor or Activity, (d) Fatigue or Inertia, (e) Depression or Dejection, and (f) Confusion or Bewilderment. Upon administering the POMS to Olympic-caliber wrestlers, rowers, and runners throughout the 1970s, Morgan graphed the results to illustrate the profiles of more and less successful athletes as compared to the general population. Because the resulting profile strongly resembled the shape of an iceberg, Morgan coined the term *Iceberg Profile* to refer to the superior emotional health of successful athletes. Specifically, more successful athletes (those who qualified for an Olympic team), tended to score higher than the general population on vigor, and lower than the general population on tension, anger, depression, fatigue, and confusion. However, less successful athletes (those who failed to qualify for an Olympic team), did not demonstrate a marked discrepancy between vigor and the other mood states. The collective results of Morgan's work led him to establish his *mental health model,* suggesting a positive association between emotional health and athletic performance.

Morgan (1979) suggested the POMS as one component of a comprehensive battery of psychological and physiological tests for athletic talent identification. More relevant to emotional health in athletes, however, was his recommendation to regularly administer the POMS to athletes to assess changes in mood due to the physical and psychological training demands of competitive sport. Morgan was one of the first to recognize the potentially deleterious influence of competitive sport on athletes' emotional health. More recent research has allowed for a more nuanced understanding of the connection between high-level sport participation and the emotional health of athletes.

Beyond the iceberg: Current status and understanding of emotional health in athletes

Although useful in beginning the discussion of emotional health in high-level athletes, Morgan's research was limited to using more broad and general measures of mental/emotional health such as the POMS rather than standardized questionnaires focused on specific emotional health issues such as depression, anxiety, disordered eating, and substance abuse. Furthermore, the notion that more elite athletes have fewer emotional health concerns than less successful athletes or non-athletes has been challenged both via scholars (e.g., Wolanin, Gross, & Hong, 2015), and via anecdotal evidence (e.g., Noren, 2014). The mainstream attention brought by stories of high-profile soccer, American football, and baseball players who experience clinical psychological disorders has raised awareness, and prompted action by sport governing bodies such as the National Collegiate Athletics Association, the English Institute of Sport, the Australian Football League, and the Canadian Olympic Committee.

A recent comprehensive review by Rice, Purcell, De Silva, Mawren, McGorry, and Parker (2016) offered insight into the prevalence and nature of emotional health concerns in elite athletes. The authors identified 60 studies meeting the stated criteria of: (a) including currently competing and able-bodied Olympic, national, international, or professional athletes; (b) reporting quantitative data on an emotional health or coping outcome; and (c) published in English. However, of the 60 studies, only about 25% met the minimum standards of "good reporting quality" (e.g., use of standardized measures, random sampling). Based on the available evidence, the authors concluded that elite athletes as a whole tend to experience emotional health issues at approximately the same rate as the general population. However, certain types of athletes seem to be more at-risk for certain disorders. For example, female athletes who compete in sports focused on leanness report higher prevalence of eating disorders than other athletes or individuals in the general population (e.g., Byrne & McLean, 2002). See Table 2.1 for a summary of selected prevalence studies on emotional health in athletes.

Thus, contrary to Morgan's contention of overall better emotional health in elite athletes, more recent investigations suggest that the issue is more complex than originally believed. Although athletes who rise to the top may do so in part because of superior emotional health, the demands and pressures inherent to competitive sport may trigger new or exacerbate existing psychopathology. Citing the intense pressure on athletes to succeed despite all odds, Bauman (2016) went so far as to suggest that the quest for mental toughness (i.e., the ability to persevere and overcome any obstacle, adversity, or pressure experienced) is incongruent with emotional health. However, Gucciardi, Hanton, and Fleming (2017) called Bauman's assertion into question, suggesting that mental toughness may represent an important component of emotional health, and as such, be used as a "hook" to facilitate conversations about emotional health in athletes. Taken together, available evidence suggests that, depending on the context, competitive sport participation can either serve as a risk or a protective factor for emotional health concerns in athletes.

Sport as a protective factor for emotional health concerns

As with cognitive health, the benefits of regular physical activity, of which sport is one form, for individuals' emotional health are well documented. For example, individuals who engage in low amounts of physical activity are significantly more likely to experience anxiety (Stubbs, Koyanagi, Hallgren, Firth, Richards, Schuch, et al., 2017), and less likely to need inpatient mental health services (Korge & Nunan, 2017). As a sub-type of physical activity, sport participation is a viable tool for enhancing emotional health and reducing emotional health

TABLE 2.1 Summary of selected prevalence studies for emotional health issues in high-level athletes

Emotional health issue	Study authors and year of publication	Participants	Measure(s)	Prevalence
Non-Performance-Specific Depression and Anxiety	Gouttebarge, Frings-Dresen, & Sluiter (2015)	301 current (M_{age} = 27 years) and former (M_{age} = 36 years) male footballers	General Health Questionnaire	26% indicated symptoms of anxiety/depression in the previous month
	Gouttebarge, Jonkers, Moen, Verhagen, Wylleman, & Kerkhoffs (2017)	203 current and 282 former elite male and female athletes from a variety of sports	General Health Questionnaire	4-week anxiety/depression prevalence of 45% for current athletes and 29% for former athletes
	Gulliver, Griffiths, Mackinnon, et al. (2015)	224 elite male and female athletes from a variety of sports (M_{age} = 24.91 years)	Center for Epidemiologic Depression Scale	27.2% reported current symptoms of major depression
	Hammond, Gialloreto, & Kubas (2013)	50 elite male and female swimmers (M_{age} = 20.5 years)	Beck Depression Inventory II, and a clinical interview based on DSM-IV TR criteria	68% of swimmers met the criteria for major depressive disorder in the previous 36 months before a major competition; 34% met criteria after the competition
	Nixdorf, Hautzinger, & Beckmann (2013)	99 elite male and female athletes from a variety of sports (M_{age} = 23.05 years)	Center for Epidemiologic Depression Scale	15% exceeded the cut-off for major depression
Clinical and Subclinical Eating Disorders	Chatterton & Petrie (2013)	732 male collegiate athletes	Questionnaire for Eating Disorder Diagnosis, seven items from the Bulimia Test-Revised	16% of athletes were symptomatic for an eating disorder; 1.1% classified as having an eating disorder

(Continued)

TABLE 2.1 Continued

Emotional health issue	Study authors and year of publication	Participants	Measure(s)	Prevalence
	DiPasquale & Petrie (2013)	146 male and 157 female collegiate athletes and age-matched non-athlete controls	Questionnaire for Eating Disorder Diagnosis	6.5% of female athletes versus 29.2% of female non-athletes were symptomatic for an eating disorder; 0.0% of female athletes versus 5.9% of female non-athletes classified as having an eating disorder; 12.2% of male athletes versus 18.2% of male non-athletes were symptomatic for an eating disorder; 0.0% of male athletes versus 0.6% of male non-athletes classified as having an eating disorder
	Martinsen & Sundgot-Borgen (2013)	611 male and female elite adolescent athletes and age-matched non-athlete controls	Eating Disorder Inventory-2 and a clinical interview based on the Eating Disorder Examination	7% of athletes versus 2.3% of non-athletes were classified as having an eating disorder, and the prevalence was higher in female athletes (14%) versus male athletes (3.2%)
	Rousselet et al. (2017)	340 high-level athletes	Eating Disorder Inventory and the Interview Grid for Multidimensional Athlete Assessment	32.9% of athletes classified as engaging in disordered eating
	Wollenberg, Shriver, & Gates (2015)	151 female collegiate athletes and age-matched non-athlete controls	Eating Attitudes Test-26	6.6% of athletes versus 16.5% of non-athletes classified as engaging in disordered eating

Substance Misuse and Abuse	Buckman, Farris, & Yusko (2013)	11,556 male collegiate athletes	Seven items regarding recency, frequency, and amount used of alcohol and other drugs among athletes self-identified as using or not using performance enhancing substances	3.1% of athletes reported using at least one performance enhancing substance (PES); 80.2% of PES users versus 68.3% of non-users reported binge drinking as typical; use of cigarettes, marijuana, cocaine, amphetamines, and narcotics was higher in PES users versus non-users
	Diehl et al. (2014)	1,138 elite adolescent athletes and age-matched non-athlete controls	Questions from the German Young Olympic Athletes' Lifestyle and Health Management Study, and the German Health Interview and Examination Survey for Children and Adolescents	84.1% of athletes versus 91.6% of non-athletes reported ever having drunk alcohol; 1.7% of athletes versus 24.4% of non-athletes reported currently smoking; 2.4% of athletes versus 16.2% of non-athletes reported consuming marijuana in last 12 months
	Strano Rossi & Botrè (2011)	100,000 urine samples collected from elite athletes aged 18 to 5 collected between 2000 and 2009	Urinalyses by anti-doping laboratories	Positive results ranged from 1.0% to 1.8% yearly (mostly stimulants, narcotics, and cannabinoids)

Sporting activity and **drug** use: Alcohol, cigarette and cannabis use among elite student **athletes**

Alcohol, Tobacco, Illicit **Drugs**, and Performance Enhancers: A Comparison of Use by College Student **Athletes** and Nonathletes concerns. In a longitudinal study of physical activity, anxiety, and depression in over 2,000 adults, Hiles, Lamers, Milaneschi, and Penninx (2017), people with diagnosed anxiety and/or depression had lower general physical activity and sport participation than healthy controls. Further, lower sport participation was associated with increased symptom severity and odds of disorder onset two years later. The authors suggested that skills and experiences central to sport, such as organization, social interaction, and opportunities for the enhancement of self-efficacy, may be particularly beneficial for emotional health.

Sport may also facilitate recovery in those with diagnosed mental illness. Carless and Douglas (2008) employed an interpretive approach to explore the process by which sport participation allowed men with serious mental illness to re-story their lives. Based on interviews with 11 men, the authors suggested that these individuals combatted the common narrative surrounding mental illness (e.g., loss of identity, social isolation, life purpose) with alternate narratives focused on action, achievement, and relationships. The authors offered various examples of how the participants re-storied according to sport:

> Interviewer: How does it make you feel when you hit the good shots?
>
> Oh, lovely yeah, feels good. You know that you can do it, like. It gives you a bit of satisfaction when you connect with the ball, when you follow through with the ball, and the club, you make contact with the ball, it's that sort of swing like, and when you know you hit it—it's that sound as well I think, you know, there's a good sound.
>
> *(p. 586)*

Galli, Reel, Henderson, and Detling (2016) found similar beliefs in disability-sport athletes, as these individuals reported a sense of appreciation and empowerment due to the work that their body could produce despite their impairment.

Thus, the available evidence suggests that competitive sport may offer both protection from the onset of emotional health concerns, as well as relief from emotional challenges related to mental and physical impairments. Of note is that studies showing a positive influence of sport on emotional health have not focused on elite competition in able-bodied competitors. The mental and physical demands of sport in these "win-at-all-costs" settings can have deleterious consequences for athletes' overall well-being, including their emotional health.

Sport as a risk factor for emotional health concerns

Along with competing in high-level sport comes the pressure for athletes to meet the performance demands set by themselves and others. Although sport participation may begin as a helpful distraction from depressive symptoms, as demands and expectations increase over time, it may exacerbate these same symptoms (Newman, Howells, & Fletcher, 2016). In addition to performance pressure, which is discussed further in Chapter 5, other common stressors encountered by high-level athletes include interpersonal/organizational conflict (e.g., Woodman & Hardy, 2010), balancing sport with other life domains (e.g., O'Neill, Allen, & Calder, 2013), and injury (e.g., Wadey, Podlog, Galli, & Mellalieu, 2016). As with non-athletes, common emotional health concerns encountered by athletes include depression, anxiety, body image concerns/disordered eating, and substance abuse. Although athletes may enter sport while already experiencing one or more emotional health concerns, these conditions may be triggered or exacerbated by their sport involvement. Specific threats to athlete psychosocial health are discussed in detail in Chapters 4–8, but suffice it to say that they can and often do have a profound influence on athletes' emotional health (Wolanin, Gross, & Hong, 2015). To counter the quotes from the study by Carless and Douglas (2008), I offer the following examples. The first quote comes from a qualitative study with collegiate divers:

> in terms of the girls having to be in their costumes and sometimes everyone is a bit body conscious and some things are said. I think that not a day goes by that I don't hear a comment in dry gym about someone not liking their body, and standing and staring in the mirror is very daily occurrence.
> *(Coyle, Gorczynski, & Gibson, 2017, p. 14)*

The second quote was drawn from a study of depression in female collegiate athletes:

> I don't think I ever knew it would be so hard to be so far from my friends and family. Not even that they were far, but that they were so far that I couldn't even drive six hours or so to see them, which I would have done. But I couldn't. I had nobody. It was a really isolating feeling.
> *(Jones, Butryn, Furst, & Semerjian, 2013)*

As the quotes suggest, when athletes feel ill-equipped to manage the demands of high-level sport, emotional health concerns may result. Indeed, despite the potential protective effects of sport on emotional health discussed previously, elite athletes experience emotional health concerns at a similar rate as non-athletes (Rice et al., 2016).

Emotional intelligence

One construct both relevant to emotional health and of recent interest to sport researchers is emotional intelligence (EI). The term was popularized by Daniel Goleman in his 1995 book of the same name, and refers to "the ability to perceive emotion, integrate emotion to facilitate thought, understand emotions, and to regulate emotions to promote personal growth" (Mayer, Salovey, & Caruso, 2004, p. 197). When examined in relation to the definition of emotional health previously described, emotional intelligence may be viewed as one expression of optimal emotional health. By contrast, individuals who experience clinical-level emotional health concerns struggle to understand and manage their emotions (Hertel, Schütz, & Lammers, 2009). Within athletes, EI has shown associations with more use of mental skills (Lane, Thelwell, Lowther, & Devonport, 2009), less competitive anxiety (Lu, Li, Hsu, & Williams, 2010), and more mental toughness (Cowden, 2016). Although there is limited research on EI and emotional health in athletes, the results of one recent study showed that EI was a significant predictor of well-being in collegiate athletes (DeFreese & Barczak, 2017).

Conclusion

Participation in high-level competitive sport offers opportunities for both the enhancement and debilitation of athletes' emotional health. Although research by Morgan in the 1970s implied that athletes had superior emotional health to non-athletes, and more successful athletes had superior emotional health than less successful athletes, research since this time supports a more complex relationship between sport and emotional health. Although the sense of competence and accomplishment derived from sport may offer relief from symptoms of emotional distress, the demands of competing in sport at a high level may promote pathological states and behaviors. Findings on EI in athletes suggest a link between this construct and performance, but further investigation is warranted to fully understand whether and how EI influences athletes' emotional health.

References

American Psychiatric Association. (2013). *Diagnostic and statistical manual of mental disorders* (5th ed.). Washington, DC: Author.

Athletic Intelligence Measures. (2017). *AIQ: Reliability and validity evidence.*

Athletic Intelligence Measures. (2018). *The AIQ will help you find hidden gems that others may overlook.* Retrieved from http://athleticintel.com/aiq/

Bauman, N. J. (2016). The stigma of mental health in athletes: are mental toughness and mental health seen as contradictory in elite sport? [Editorial]. *British Journal of Sports Medicine, 50*(3), 135–136. doi:10.1136/bjsports-2015-095570

Beidler, E., Bretzin, A., Hancock, C., & Covassin, T. (2017). Sport-related concussion knowledge and reporting behaviors of collegiate club sport athletes. *Journal of Athletic Training, 52*(6), S232. doi:10.4085/1062-6050-266-17

beyondblue. (n.d.). *What is mental health?* Retrieved from https://www.beyondblue.org.au/the-facts/what-is-mental-health

Buckman, J. F., Farris, S. G., & Yusko, D. A. (2013). A national study of substance use behaviors among NCAA male athletes who use banned performance enhancing substances. *Drug and Alcohol Dependence, 131*(1–2), 50–55. doi:10.1016/j.drugalcdep.2013.04.023

Byrne, S., & McLean, N. (2002). Elite athletes: Effects of the pressure to be thin. *Journal of Science and Medicine in Sport, 5*(2), 80–94. doi:10.1016/S1440-2440(02)80029-9

Canadian Mental Health Association. (2015). *What's the difference between mental health and mental illness?* Retrieved from www.heretohelp.bc.ca/ask-us/whats-the-difference-between-mental-health-and-mental-illness

Carless, D., & Douglas, K. (2008). Narrative, identity and mental health: How men with serious mental illness re-story their lives through sport and exercise. *Psychology of Sport and Exercise, 9*(5), 576–594. doi:10.1016/j.psychsport.2007.08.002

Carroll, J. B. (2003). The higher-stratum structure of cognitive abilities: Current evidence supports g and about ten broad factors. In H. Nyborg (Ed.), *The scientific study of general intelligence: Tribute to Arthur R. Jensen* (pp. 5–22). San Diego, CA: Pergamon.

Chaddock, L., Neidere, M. B., Voss, M. W., Gaspar, J. G., & Kramer, A. F. (2011). Do athletes excel at everyday tasks? *Medicine & Science in Sports & Exercise, 43*(10), 1920–1926. doi:10.1249/MSS.0b013e318218ca74

Chatterton, J. M., & Petrie, T. A. (2013). Prevalence of disordered eating and pathogenic weight control behaviors among male collegiate athletes. *Eating Disorders, 21*(4), 328–341, doi:10.1080/10640266.2013.797822

Coakley, J. (1992). Burnout among adolescent athletes: A personal failure or social problem. *Sociology of Sport Journal, 9*, 271–285. doi:10.1123/ssj.9.3.271

Cowden, R. G. (2016). Mental toughness, emotional intelligence, and coping effectiveness: An analysis of construct interrelatedness among high-performing adolescent male athletes. *Perceptual and Motor Skills, 123*(3), 737–753. https://doi.org/10.1177/0031512516666027

Coyle, M., Gorczynski, P., & Gibson, K. (2017). "You have to be mental to jump off a board any way": Elite divers' conceptualizations and perceptions of mental health. *Psychology of Sport and Exercise, 29*, 10–18. doi:10.1016/j.psychsport.2016.11.005

DeFreese, J. D., & Barczak, N. (2017). A pilot study of trait emotional intelligence as a moderator of the associations among social perceptions, athlete burnout, and well-being in collegiate athletes. *Athletic Training and Sports Health Care, 9*(6), 246–253. doi:10.3928/19425864-20171010-01

Delaney, J. S., Lamfookon, C., Bloom, G. A., Al-Kashmiri, A., & Correa J. A. (2015). Why university athletes choose not to reveal their concussion symptoms during a practice or game. *Clinical Journal of Sport Medicine, 25*(2), 113–25. doi:10.1097/JSM.0000000000000112 doi:10.1097/JSM.0000000000000112

Diehl, K., Thiel, A., Zipfel, S., Mayer, J., & Schneider, S. (2014). Risk behavior among elite adolescent athletes. *Scandinavian Journal of Medicine & Science in Sports, 24*, 250–258. doi:10.1111/j.1600-0838.2012.01472.x

DiPasquale, L. D., & Petrie, T. A. (2013). Prevalence of disordered eating: A comparison of male and female collegiate athletes and nonathletes. *Journal of Clinical Sport Psychology, 7*(3), 186–197. doi:10.1123/jcsp.7.3.186

Faubert, J. (2013). Professional athletes have extraordinary skills for rapidly learning complex and neutral dynamic visual scenes. *Scientific Reports, 3*, 1154. doi:10.1038/srep01154

Galli, N., Reel, J. J., Henderson, H., & Detling, N. (2016). An investigation of body image in athletes with physical disabilities. *Journal of Clinical Sport Psychology, 10*(1), 1–18. doi:10.1123/JCSP.2015-0018

García-Hermoso, A., Ramírez-Vélez, R., Celis-Morales, C. A., Olloquequi, J., & lIzquierdo, M. (2018). Can physical activity attenuate the negative association between sitting time and cognitive function among older adults? A mediation analysis. *Experimental Gerontology, 106*, 173–177. doi:10.1016/j.exger.2018.03.002

Gerrig, R. J. (2012). *Psychology and life* (20th ed.). Boston, MA: Pearson Higher Education.

Ginsburg, K. R. (2007). The importance of play in promoting healthy child development and maintaining strong parent–child bonds. *Pediatrics, 119*(1), 182–191. doi:10.1542/peds.2006-2697

Gouttebarge, V., Frings-Dresen, M. H. W., & Sluiter, J. K. (2015). Mental and psychosocial health among current and former professional footballers. *Occupational Medicine, 65*(3), 190–196. doi:10.1093/occmed/kqu202

Gouttebarge, V., Jonkers, R., Moen, M., Verhagen, E., Wylleman, P., & Kerkhoffs, G. (2017). The prevalence and risk indicators of symptoms of common mental disorders among current and former Dutch elite athletes. *Journal of Sports Sciences, 35,* 2148–2156. doi:10.1080/02640414.2016.1258485

Gucciardi, D., Hanton, S., & Fleming, S. (2017). Are mental toughness and mental health contradictory concepts in elite sport? A narrative review of theory and evidence. *Journal of Science and Medicine in Sport. 20*(3), 307–311. doi:10.1016/j.jsams.2016.08.006

Gulliver, A., Griffiths, K. M., Mackinnon, A., Batterham, P. J., & Stanimirovic, R. (2015). The mental health of Australian elite athletes. *Journal of Science and Medicine in Sport, 18*(3), 255–261. doi:10.1016/j.jsams.2014.04.006

Hammond, T., Gialloreto, C., Kubas, H., & Davis, H. (2013). The prevalence of failure-based depression among elite athletes. *Clinical Journal of Sport Medicine, 23*(4), 273–277. doi:10.1097/JSM.0b013e318287b870

Harvard Medical School. (2017). *Data Table 2: 12-month prevalence of DSM-IV/WMH-CIDI disorders by sex and cohort* (National Comorbidity Survey). Retrieved from https://www.hcp.med.harvard.edu/ncs/ftpdir/table_ncsr_12monthprevgenderxage.pdf

Hertel, J., Schütz, A., & Lammers, C.-H. (2009). Emotional intelligence and mental disorder. *Journal of Clinical Psychology, 65*(9), 942–954. doi:10.1002/jclp.20597

Hiles, S. A., Lamers, F., Milaneschi, Y., & Penninx, B. W. J. H. (2017). Sit, step, sweat: Longitudinal associations between physical activity patterns, anxiety and depression. *Psychological Medicine, 47*(8), 1466–1477. doi:10.1017/S0033291716003548

Jones, A., Butryn, T. M., Furst, D. M., & Semerjian, T. Z. (2013). A phenomenological examination of depression in female Division-I athletes. *Athletic Insight: The Online Journal of Sport Psychology, 5,* 1-19. doi:10.1016/j.psychsport.2016.11.005

Korge, J., & Nunan, D. (2017). Higher participation in physical activity is associated with less use of inpatient mental health services: A cross-sectional study. *Psychiatry Research,* 259, 550–553 doi:10.1016/j.psychres.2017.11.030

Lane, A. M., Thelwell, R. C., Lowther, J., & Devonport, T. J. (2009). Emotional intelligence and psychological skills use among athletes. *Social Behavior and Personality: An International Journal, 37*(2), 195–201. doi:10.2224/sbp.2009.37.2.195

Langlois, J. A., Rutland-Brown, W., & Wald, M. M. (2006). The epidemiology and impact of traumatic brain injury: A brief overview. *Journal of Head Trauma Rehabilitation, 21*(5), 375–378.

Lu, F. J.-H., Li, G. S-F., Hsu, E. Y-W., & Williams, L. (2010). Relationship between athletes' emotional intelligence and precompetitive anxiety. *Perceptual and Motor Skills, 110*(1), 323–338. doi:10.2466/pms.110.1.323-338

Lyons, B. D., Hoffman, B. J., & Michel, J. W. (2009). Not much more than *g*? An examination of the impact of intelligence on NFL performance. *Human Performance, 22*(3), 225–245. doi:10.1080/08959280902970401

Martinsen, M., & Sundgot-Borgen, J. (2013). Higher prevalence of eating disorders among adolescent elite athletes than controls. *Medicine & Science in Sports & Exercise, 45,* 1188–1197. doi:10.1249/MSS.0b013e318281a939

Mayer, J. D., Salovey, P., & Caruso, D. R. (2004). Emotional intelligence: Theory, findings, and implications. *Psychological Inquiry, 15,* 197-215. doi:10.1207/s15327965pli1503_02

Mayo Clinic. (2018). *Depression (major depressive disorder).* Retrieved from https://www.mayoclinic.org/diseases-conditions/depression/symptoms-causes/syc-20356007

McBride, R. E., & Reed, J. (1998). Thinking and college athletes—Are they predisposed to critical thinking? *College Student Journal, 32*(3), 443.

McNair, D., Lorr, M., & Doppleman, L. (1971). *POMS manual for the profile of mood states.* San Diego, CA: Educational and Industrial Testing Service.

Moore, R. D., Hillman, C. H., & Broglio, S. P. (2014). The persistent influence of concussive injuries on cognitive control and neuroelectric function. *Journal of Athletic Training, 49*(1), 24–35. doi:10.4085/1062-6050-49.1.01

Morgan, W. P. (1979). Prediction of performance in athletics. In P. Klavora & J. V. Daniel (Eds.), *Coach, athlete, and the sport psychologist* (pp. 173–186). Champaign, IL: Human Kinetics.

National Institute of Neurological Disorders and Stroke, National Institute of Mental Health, & National Institute of Aging. (2001). *Cognitive and emotional health: The Healthy Brain Workshop.* Retrieved from https://trans.nih.gov/CEHP/NINDSSummary.pdf

Newman, H. J. H., Howells, K. L., & Fletcher, D. (2016). The dark side of top level sport: An autobiographic study of depressive experiences in elite sport performers. *Frontiers in Psychology, 7,* 868. doi:10.3389/fpsyg.2016.00868

Nixdorf, I., Frank, R., Hautzinger, M., & Beckmann, J. (2013). Prevalence of depressive symptoms and correlating variables among German elite athletes. Journal of Clinical Sport Psychology, 7(4), 313–326. doi:10.1123/jcsp.7.4.313

Noren, N. (2014). *Taking notice of the hidden injury.* Retrieved from www.espn.com/espn/otl/story/_/id/10335925/awareness-better-treatment-college-athletes-mental-health-begins-take-shape

O'Neill, M., Allen, B., & Calder, A. M. (2013). Pressures to perform: An interview study of Australian high performance school-age athletes' perceptions of balancing their school and sporting lives. *Performance Enhancement and Health, 2*(3), 87–93. doi:10.1016/j.peh.2013.06.001

Peretti-Watel, P., Guagliardo, V., Verger, P., Pruvost, J., Mignon, P., & Obadia, Y. (2003). Sporting activity and drug use: Alcohol, cigarette and cannabis use among elite student athletes. *Addiction, 98,* 1249–1256. doi:10.1046/j.1360-0443.2003.00490.x

Pittsburgh's Action News 4. (2017, May 2). *Sidney Crosby has concussion, ruled out for Penguins–Capitals game 4.* Retrieved from https://www.wtae.com/article/penguins-sidney-crosby-leaves-following-hit-to-head/9589921

Rice, S. M., Purcell, R., De Silva, S., Mawren, D., McGorry, P. D., & Parker, A. G. (2016). The mental health of elite athletes: A narrative systematic review. *Sports Medicine, 46*(9), 1333–1353. doi:10.1007/s40279-016-0492-2

Rousselet, M., Guérineau, B., Paruit, M. C., Guinot, M., Lise, S., Destrube, B., … Prétagut, S. (2017). Disordered eating in French high-level athletes: Association with type of sport, doping behavior, and psychological features. *Eating and Weight Disorders, 22,* 61. doi:10.1007/s40519-016-0342-0

Schurr, K. T., Ashley, M. A., & Joy, K. L. (1977). A multivariate analysis of male athlete personality characteristics: Sport type and success. *Multivariate Experimental Clinical Research, 3*(2), 53–68.

Simons, H. D., Bosworth, C., Fujita, S., & Jensen, M. (2007). The athlete stigma in higher education. *College Student Journal, 41,* 251–273.

Singh-Manoux, A., Kivimaki, M., Glymour, M. M., Elbaz, A., Berr, C., Ebmeier, K. P., … Dugravot, A. (2012). Timing of onset of cognitive decline: Results from Whitehall II prospective cohort study. *BMJ.* doi:10.1136/bmj.d7622

Slusher, H. S. (1964). Personality and intelligence characteristics of selected high school athletes and nonathletes. *Research Quarterly, 35,* 539–545. doi:10.1080/10671188.1964.10613351

Stice, E., & Bohon, C. (2013). Eating disorders. In T. Beauchaine & S. Linshaw (Eds.), *Child and adolescent psychopathology* (2nd ed., pp. 715–738). New York, NY: Wiley.

Strano Rossi, S., & Botrè, F. (2011). Prevalence of illicit drug use among the Italian athlete population with special attention on drugs of abuse: A 10-year review. *Journal of Sports Sciences, 29*(5), 471–476. doi:10.1080/02640414.2010.543915

Stubbs, B., Koyanagi, A., Hallgren, M., Firth, J., Richards, J., Schuch, F., ... Vancampfort, D. (2017). Physical activity and anxiety: A perspective from the World Health Survey. *Journal of Affective Disorders, 208*, 545–552. doi:10.1016/j.jad.2016.10.028

Substance Abuse and Mental Health Services Administration. (2015a). *Mental disorders.* Retrieved from https://www.samhsa.gov/disorders/mental

Substance Abuse and Mental Health Services Administration. (2015b). *Substance use disorders.* Retrieved from https://www.samhsa.gov/disorders/substance-use

Tseng, B. Y., Uh, J., Rossetti, H. C., Cullum, M., Diaz-Arrastia, R. F., Levine, B. D., ... Zhang, R. (2013). Masters athletes exhibit larger regional brain volume and better cognitive performance than sedentary older adults. *Journal of Magnetic Resonance Imaging, 38*(5). doi:10.1002/jmri.24085

Wade, C., & Tavris, C. (1998). *Psychology.* Harlow, United Kingdom: Longman.

Wadey, R., Podlog, L., Galli, N., & Mellalieu, S. D. (2016). Stress-related growth following sport injury: Examining the applicability of the organismic valuing theory. *Scandinavian Journal of Medicine & Science in Sports, 26*(10), 1132–1139. doi:10.1111/sms.12579

Williams, A. M., & Ericsson, K. A. (2005). Some considerations when applying the expert performance approach in sport. *Human Movement Science, 24*, 283–307.

Winenger, S. R., & White, T. A. (2015). An examination of the dumb jock stereotype in collegiate student-athletes: A comparison of student versus student-athlete perceptions. *Journal for the Study of Sports and Athletes in Education, 9*(2), 75–85. doi:10.1179/1935739715Z.00000000036

Wolanin, A., Gross, M., & Hong, E. (2015). Depression in athletes: Prevalence and risk factors. *Current Sports Medicine Reports, 14*, 56–60. doi:10.1249/JSR.0000000000000123

Wollenberg. G., Shriver, L. H., & Gates, G. E. (2015). Comparison of disordered eating symptoms and emotion regulation difficulties between female college athletes and non-athletes. *Eating Behaviors, 18*, 1–6. doi:10.1016/j.eatbeh.2015.03.008

Wonderlic, E. F., & Hovland, C. I. (1939). The Personnel Test: A restandardized abridgment of the Otis S-A test for business and industrial use. *Journal of Applied Psychology, 23*(6), 685–702. doi:10.1037/h0056432

Woodman, T., & Hardy, L. (2010). A case study of organizational stress in elite sport. *Journal of Applied Sport Psychology, 13*(2), 207–238, doi:10.1080/104132001753149892

World Health Organization. (2014). Mental health: A state of well-being. Retrieved from https://www.who.int/features/factfiles/mental_health/en/

Yusko, D. A., Buckman, J. F., White, H. R., & Pandina, R. J. (2008). Alcohol, tobacco, illicit drugs, and performance enhancers: A comparison of use by college student athletes and nonathletes. *Journal of American College Health, 57*(3), 281–290. doi:10.3200/JACH.57.3.281-290

3

SOCIAL AND SPIRITUAL HEALTH

Emil is in his first season as a starting midfielder for his national football team. His first season has gone remarkably well both in terms of his relationships with teammates and coaches, as well as the team's on-field performance. Emil is a faithful Muslim and observes Ramadan every year by abstaining from food and liquids from sunrise until sunset every day for an entire month. This year, Ramadan occurs during June, which also happens to be at the same time as the European Championship tournament. Upon notifying his coaches, Emil notices a change in how his coaches interact with and choose to deploy him. Although Emil feels that he is balancing his fasting and training well, the coaches begin noticeably conversing about him on the sideline during practice. They off-hand suggestions to him that he make up his fasting during another time of the year as "other athletes have done." Finally, the head coach discusses reducing his minutes during the tournament, claiming that he seems "a step slow," and is concerned about him "running out of steam" during matches. Emil is hurt by all of this, and feels that he is being unfairly treated due to his spiritual beliefs. Not only does he feel confident in his level of conditioning, but has always considered his faith to be an important part of what drives him as a player. In turn, his training serves to reinforce his beliefs. Now, the spiritual doctrine that he has grown up with seems to be working against him. The one bright spot is that Emil's teammates are aware of the situation, and remain incredibly supportive during this time.

The preceding scenario illustrates the intersection of the two outer-rings of psychosocial health for athletes—social and spiritual health (Figure 1.1). As opposed to the cognitive and emotional dimensions of health, the social and spiritual dimensions reflect athletes' connection with outside forces. In this chapter I introduce these two dimensions of health, and consider their relevance for high-level sport participation.

Social health

Social health refers to the degree to which individuals can effectively interact with others, use social support, and adapt to various social situations (Donatelle, 2014). As mentioned in Chapter 1, the social dimension of health, often referred to as social well-being, includes the degree to which individuals feel integrated into society (i.e., social integration), trust and accept others (i.e., social acceptance), contribute to society (i.e., social contribution), feel hopeful about the future of society (i.e., social actualization), and believe that they can make sense of the world around them (i.e., social coherence) (Keyes, 1998). Within sport, the social dimension of health can be examined both in terms of its influence on athletes' general interpersonal functioning (i.e., prosocial behavior) and in terms of athletes' social functioning within the sport environment.

Although much has been written about the social dimension of health as it relates to motivation and prosocial behavior within youth sport and physical activity (e.g., Bruner, Boardley, Benson, Wilson, Root, Turnnidge, Sutcliffe, & Côté, 2017; Stuntz & Weiss, 2009), social health and well-being within high-level adult sport has largely been ignored. Two relatively recent qualitative studies are exceptions. The first, by Lundqvist and Sandin (2014), was conducted to better understand holistic (i.e., hedonic, eudaimonic, global, contextual) well-being in elite male and female orienteers (median age = 20.4 years). Semi-structured interviews followed by content analysis revealed several insights relevant to social health. Positive relations with others both in and out of sport were reported as important parts of orienteers' well-being. The availability of social support in the form of friends and family were served not only as an important coping strategy when faced with obstacles within sport, but also a welcome distraction from the rigors of training and competition. Within sport, quality support from coaches and peers were perceived by athletes as vital for personal and athletic development. Related specifically to Keyes' dimensions of social well-being, the athletes discussed social coherence as represented by unconditional positive regard from teammates. Another interesting finding related to social health was athletes' recognition of positive qualities and successes of other competitors (Lundqvist & Sandin, 2014).

A second study, by Macdougall, O'Halloran, Sherry, and Shields (2016), focused on well-being in Australian Para-athletes. Data were gathered through a combination of one-on-one interviews and focus groups with 23 male and female athletes from a variety of sports (M_{age} = 28.5 years). Similar to Lundqvist and Sandin (2014), the researchers identified aspects of social health and well-being affecting athletes at both the global and sport-specific levels. However, Macdougall et al. went further to identify both social strengths and needs of the athletes. For example, athletes identified a need for progress in terms of social actualization and integration due to pervasive and limiting societal stereotypes about physical disability, as well as the perception that mental health issues remained a taboo subject within their team. By contrast, athletes noted considerable social contribution benefits of sport participation, including the opportunity to volunteer in the community, and with youth at lower levels of the sport.

The results of the aforementioned studies offer some insight into the social health experiences of high-level athletes. However, much work clearly remains to gain a complete understanding of the antecedents, consequences, and sport-specific aspects of social health and well-being for high-level athletes. As noted by Lundqvist and Sandin (2014), the age of athletes included in typical studies of high-level athletes may be a limiting factor, as social well-being may increase with age (Keyes, 1998). As previously mentioned, one construct that has received considerable attention in sport, and that seemingly reflects the acceptance and integration elements of social well-being, is social support.

Because competitive sports are by nature a social endeavor in which individuals often form close interpersonal relationships with teammates and coaches, they offer an ideal setting for athletes to give and receive support from others (Wylleman, 2000). For example, in 2012, the two-year-old daughter of Rory Otto, a former swimmer for Princeton University, was diagnosed with a rare and debilitating disease known as Fibrodysplasia Ossificans Progressiva, in which bone forms within soft tissue (Chadeayne, 2012). Members of the current team put on a fundraiser resulting in $62,000 for Otto. Support can also be intangible. Following the Canadian Women's Ice Hockey team's loss in the gold medal game at the 2018 Winter Olympics, fellow Olympians took to social media to offer their support through messages such as "Breaks my heart to see these incredible women look sad getting their silver medals! You all played so amazing and Canada is incredibly proud of you!" (Francois, 2018). In the next sections I offer an overview of social support in general, followed by a summary of research specific to social support in high-level athletes.

Social support

First formally studied in the realm of preventive medicine, *social support* refers to "information leading the subject to believe that he is cared for and loved, esteemed, and a member of a network of mutual obligations" (Cobb, 1976, p. 300). Although a variety of sub-types/functions of social support have been suggested, the four most common functions of social support discussed in the literature are *emotional* (e.g., the offering of empathy or compassion), *tangible* (e.g., provision of financial assistance or helpful services), *informational* (e.g., advice, counseling), and *companionship* (e.g., sense of belonging with others) (Wills, 1991). Three dimensions are considered when examining social support: (a) *structural* (i.e., who is providing support), (b) *functional* (how the support is provided), and (c) *perceptual* (i.e., subjective perceptions of availability and quality of support) (Wills, O'Carroll Bantum, & Ainette, 2016). Further distinctions are made between *perceived* (i.e., individuals' subjective belief that support has been given or offered) and *received* (i.e., objective assistance provided) social support (Helgeson, 1993). In non-sport research, perceived support has shown stronger relationships with positive outcomes such as facilitative coping compared to received support (Uchino, 2009). Various theories have been proposed to explain the positive influence of social support on overall health, including the stress and coping theory, relational regulation theory, and life-span theory (Lakey, 2010). Overall, these theories suggest mechanisms through which perceived and/or received social support act as a buffer to stress and/or promote adaptive emotional regulation enhancing mental health.

Social support in sport

Despite a plethora of studies involving social support in general psychology in the 1970s and 1980s, it was not until 1989 that the first study on social support in high-level athletes was published. In this study, Rosenfeld, Richman, and Hardy (1989) examined the type and amount of perceived social support offered to high- and low-stressed collegiate athletes. A unique aspect of this study was the inclusion of sport-specific types of social support—technical challenge (i.e., encouraging athletes to achieve more), and technical appreciation (i.e., acknowledgment of successful performance). Using a mixed-methods approach involving both self-report questionnaire data and interviews with athletes and coaches, the authors found that *shared social reality,* characterized by interactions with others who have similar experiences and serve as a reality check, was the most frequently cited type of social support perceived. Differences in the type of support offered depending on the source were also found. Whereas coaches and teammates tended to support challenging athletes to achieve more, parents and friends tended to offer more emotional and listening support.

The Rosenfeld et al. (1989) study is notable for being the first focused on social support in high-level athletes. Since 1989 many more peer-reviewed articles on the topic have been published, often focused on social support in the context of athletic injury (e.g., Johnston & Carroll, 1998; Udry, 1997; Yang, Peek-Asa, Lowe, Heiden, & Foster, 2010). Research suggests that not all social support is created equal for injured athletes (Fernandes, Reis, Vilaca-Alves, Saavedra, Aidar, & Brustad, 2014). Depending on the stage of recovery, injured athletes have noted a preference for different types of support and from different sources. For example, when athletes are preparing to return to competition, informational support from medical professionals and coaches is most important.

A systematic review of studies on social support in youth athletes (including elite athletes up to the age of 22) by Sheridan, Coffee, and Lavallee (2014) offers a current perspective on social support for athletes across a variety of situations. Not surprisingly, social support (or lack thereof) from sources both within and outside of sport were found to have a powerful effect on athletes' motivation, level of achievement, and overall sport experience. Further, the findings largely support those of Rosenfeld et al.'s (1989) seminal work, in that coaches are the most frequent and powerful social support provider. For example, Le Bars, Gernigon, and Ninot (2009) found that athletes viewed the creation of a task-oriented climate by coaches as helpful in their transition to elite sport. Jowett (e.g., Jowett, 2017; Jowett & Cockerill, 2003) has written extensively on the coach-athlete relationship, and noted 3 C's characterizing coach-athlete dyads: (a) Closeness (e.g., trust and respect), (b) Co-orientation (e.g., shared goals), and (c) Complementarity (e.g., the interplay between coach feedback and athlete coachability). In one of the early studies in this area, Jowett and Cockerill noted the presence of all 3 C's (in both positive and negative directions) in interviews with 12 Olympic medalists regarding their coach relationships. Thus, although more work remains, social support, and particularly support provided as part of the coach-athlete relationship, represents the most well-understood indicator of athletes' social health and well-being.

Summary

Although the social dimension of health has garnered much attention in the realm of youth sport, much less research has been conducted on the social health of high-level adult athletes. Only two studies have specifically included an examination of social well-being in samples of non-youth athletes. Work on social support, which partially reflects social well-being, is more prominent, and findings from studies of social support in high-level athletes suggest the simultaneous consideration of the type, source, and timing for athletes. Coaches have emerged as a critical source of support, and may well be the primary influence on high-level athletes' social health.

Spiritual health

Of the four dimensions of health addressed in this text, spiritual health is the most recently recognized, and perhaps the most controversial. Prior to 1984, the World Health Organization (WHO) recognized only the physical, social, and mental/emotional dimensions of health (WHO, 1998). In 1983, delegates from several Middle Eastern countries, including Bahrain, Iraq, and Kuwait, proposed greater emphasis on the spiritual dimension of health. Resolution WHA31.13 was passed in 1984 by the 37th WHO World Health Assembly, and recommends that all WHO members consider spiritual health in concordance with their personal Health For All initiative. Even before resolution WHA31.13, health education scholars called for a focus on the spiritual dimension of health (e.g., Banks, 1980; Young, 1984). In response to growing concerns about the operationalization and measurement of the spiritual dimension of health, Hawks (1994) brought some clarity to the issue by offering a working definition of spiritual health. Based on extant literature, Hawks defined *spiritual health* as "A high level of faith, hope, and commitment in relation to a well-defined worldview or belief system that provides a sense of meaning and purpose to existence in general, and that offers an ethical path to personal fulfillment which includes connectedness with self, others, and a higher power or larger reality" (p. 7). Because of its emphasis on a sense of meaning and purpose, spiritual health seems closely related to Ryff's (1989) conception of PWB. Indeed, research supports the association between spiritual health and PWB in young adults and adolescents (Burney, Osmany, & Khan, 2017; Kumar, 2015). Hawks further explained the two major ways in which spiritual health is studied: (a) the intrinsic characteristics of people who are spiritually well (e.g., life purpose, connectedness with others), and (b) how spiritually well people express themselves to and with others (e.g., trust, honesty, compassion). Research conducted since Hawks' seminal article has established relationships between spiritual health and a variety of facilitative outcomes and characteristics, including higher quality of life (Yaghobi, Abdekhoda, & Khani, 2018), better emotional regulation (Jamali, Shakerina, Nikoo, & Jobaneh, 2017), less depression (Jafari, Ebad, Rezaei, & Ashtarian, 2017), and higher self-esteem (Abbasian, Kia, Mirmohammadkhani, Gharemanfard, & Ghods, 2016).

Despite the upsurge of interest in the spiritual dimension of health since the 1980s, scholars of high-level sport have not displayed similar enthusiasm for the area. Such lack of interest is slightly perplexing, as many high-profile athletes have openly cited their spirituality, in the form of religion, as a driving force, and attributed their successes to a higher power (Lee, 2011). Perhaps the most famous recent example in the U.S. is former American football and current baseball player Tim Tebow, who famously made a habit of kneeling in prayer (i.e., "Tebowing") during football games, and often wrote Bible verses on his eye black tape. In a recent *Sports Illustrated* article, Clayton Kershaw of Major League Baseball's Los Angeles Dodgers spoke of how he views every failure as an affront to the God who bestowed him with his talent (Apstein, 2018). The research that has been conducted in high-level sport has focused on spirituality in the form of religion, which is "a personal set or institutionalized system of attitudes, beliefs, and practices related to an acknowledged ultimate deity" (Merriam-Webster, 2018), and its link to athlete preparation and performance, rather than on spiritual health specifically. In the following section I review the literature on spirituality, religion, and the sport experience of high-level athletes, including a focus on the recent work related to mindfulness.

Spirituality and religion in high-level athletes

Early research compared the spirituality and/or religiousness of athletes and non-athletes. As part of their line of inquiry on multidimensional self-concept, Marsh, Perry, Horsely, and Roche (1995) found that non-athletes scored significantly higher on the *Spiritual Values/Religion* subscale of the Self-Description Questionnaire for late adolescents and young adults. Storch, Kolsky, Silvestri, and Storch (2001) focused more specifically on religiousness in their comparison of

Division I collegiate athletes and non-athletes. The authors employed the Duke Religion Index (DRI; Koenig, Parkerson, & Meador, 1997) to measure both groups on three dimensions of religiousness: (a) organizational (e.g., attending church services), (b) non-organizational (e.g., personal prayer), and (c) intrinsic (e.g., internalization of religion as an essential part of one's self-identity). The findings revealed a gender × sport status interaction, such that male non-athletes reported significantly lower religiousness on all three dimensions of the construct. The authors emphasized that athletes reported only a mild to moderate degree of religiousness. Storch et al. (Storch, Roberti, Bravata, & Storch, 2004) followed up the 2001 study with a second one comparing collegiate athletes and non-athletes, this time using the Santa Clara Strength of Religious Faith Questionnaire-Short Form (SCFRFQ-SF; Plante, Vallaeys, Sherman, & Wallston, 2002). Once again, although the overall mean score indicated only moderately strong religious faith, athletes scored significantly higher than non-athletes. Bell, Johnson, and Petersen (2009) considered the type of institution (religiously-practicing versus non-religiously practicing) into their investigation of religious faith in athletes and non-athletes. Athletes at religiously-practicing institutions scored significantly lower on strength of religious faith than non-athletes at the same institutions. Thus, despite oft-publicized expressions of spirituality by mainstream athletes, the available research suggests that athletes are at most only marginally more religious/spiritual than non-athletes, and in some cases, as in the investigation by Bell et al., less so.

Questionnaire-based examinations of religiousness and spirituality such as those previously described ignore the subjective meanings and experiences of athletes who identify as being religious or spiritual. Qualitative investigations have added depth to our understanding of the role of religion and spirituality for high-level athletes, and perhaps offer greater insight into their spiritual health. Ravizza's (1977) seminal study was the first to elicit athletes' subjective experience of their greatest moment in sports. In interviews with 20 athletes, peak experience was characterized by several qualities, including loss of fear, a feeling of Godlike control, transcendence of ordinary self, and awe and wonder. Regarding transcendence, a skier noted how they "blended into the snow" during their peak experience. In the implications section of his article. Ravizza noted that the results of his study gave credence to the importance of cognition and emotion in athletes' sport experience. I argue that the stories told by these athletes are also suggestive of the potential for sport to trigger moments of optimal spiritual health. Subsequent qualitative investigations of *flow*—a state in which individuals are fully immersed in an enjoyable activity (Csikszentmihályi, 1990)—further support competitive sport as an ideal site for the experience of personal connection to a "larger reality," which is inherent to spiritual health (e.g., Russell, 2001). A study by Galli and Reel (2012) highlights another way in which high-level sport may enhance spiritual health—through the experience of adversity. Interviews with high-level athletes from a variety of sports on the psychosocial consequences of their most difficult sport adversity revealed that many of the athletes perceived spiritual enhancement due to their experience. The following quote from a track and field athlete illustrates her perceptions of spiritual change due to a serious automobile accident:

> I feel like I need to be a vessel for God in some aspects, and we've been going to church together and kind of growing not only physically together but also spiritually and obviously emotionally since we go through the pr's and all the good things you do and the meets where you just do horrible.
>
> *(p. 14)*

Other studies have gone beyond exploring the spiritual experiences of high-level athletes to examine the link between spirituality and other indices of health and well-being. Storch et al. (e.g., Storch, Kovacs, Roberti, Bailey, Bravata, & Storch, 2004) are responsible for much of the work establishing links between religiousness and indicators of emotional and social health, including depression (Storch, Storch, Welsh, & Okun, 2002), substance abuse (Storch, Storch, Kovacs, Okun, & Welsh, 2003), social anxiety (Storch, Storch, & Adams, 2002), social support (Storch & Storch, 2002), aggression (Storch & Storch, 2002), and overall psychological adjustment (Storch et al., 2004) in intercollegiate athletes. The results of these studies were mixed, as no significant correlations between religiousness and social anxiety, social support, or indices of psychological adjustment emerged. However, the researchers did find significant inverse correlations between intrinsic religiousness and depression, substance abuse, and aggression. In support of the latter, other researchers have found religiousness to be a protective factor for unhealthy behaviors such as alcohol use, sexual activity, use of appetite suppressants, and hesitancy to dope in collegiate athletes (Cavar, Sekulic, & Culjak, 2012; Moore, Berkley-Patton, and Hawes, 2013; Zenic, Stipic, & Sekulic, 2013). Thus, there is some evidence that greater spiritual health, as measured by the strength of religious faith, is related to healthier behaviors and better emotional health. Of note is the cross-sectional design adopted in these studies, which precludes causal inference.

More so than the cognitive, emotional, and social dimensions of psychosocial health, the spiritual dimension is strongly linked to cultural identification. The connection between spiritual health and sport may be particularly strong in Eastern cultures, where collectivism is valued over independent achievement, and connection with the world/universe is more central to individuals' experience. In one study, the attitudes toward sport of student-athletes at a Japanese university were examined in relation to whether they participated in English-based (e.g., tennis), American-based (e.g., American football), or Japanese-based (e.g., Kendo) sports. As opposed to the participants in English-based sports, who valued sportsmanship, and participants in American-based sports, who most valued traits such as victory and power, individuals who competed in traditional Japanese sports viewed participation as being essential for spiritual cultivation (Niwa, 1993). At times, the win-at-all-costs culture of sport can clash with high-level athletes' spiritual and religious beliefs. The following quote from a qualitative study of the challenges encountered by African athletes competing at U.S. universities illustrates this conflict:

> Man I don't even want to tell people that I am Muslim anymore … What if [I was] Hindu? Sometimes my coach doesn't want me to fast during Ramadan. This is like telling me, 'Don't practice your religious beliefs.'
>
> *(Lee & Opio, 2011, p. 637)*

Dispositional mindfulness in high-level athletes

A spiritually rooted concept that has recently garnered attention from sport scholars and practitioners is *mindfulness*, defined by Kabat-Zinn (1994) as present-moment awareness that is both purposeful and non-judgmental. Mindfulness is the American translation of the term *Sati,* which is the first of the Seven Factors of Enlightenment in Buddhism (Carmody, Reed, Kristeller, & Merriam, 2008). Although several investigations have focused solely on the use of mindfulness *practices* (i.e., cultivated mindfulness; Baer, Smith, Hopkins, Krietemeyer, & Toney, 2006) to enhance well-being and performance in high-level athletes, others have examined relations between athletes' well-being and their general tendency to exhibit nonjudgmental and nonreactive awareness of thoughts, emotions, and present moment experience (i.e., dispositional mindfulness; Baer et al., 2006). For example, Moen, Federici, and Abrahamsen (2015) examined the links between self-reported mindfulness, stress, and burnout in 483 elite junior Norwegian athletes. As expected, mindfulness was negatively related to both perceptions of stress and burnout. Similarly, Gustafsson, Skoog, Davis, Kenttä, and Haberl (2015) found negative relationships between dispositional mindfulness, stress, and burnout in elite junior athletes, and that these relationships were mediated by affect. For young adult athletes, mindfulness has been linked to lower stress, better coping, and the tendency to experience flow states during performance (Cathcart, McGregor, & Groundwater, 2014; Kaiseler, Poolton, Backhouse, & Stanger, 2017).

Thus, as in non-athletes, extant research supports dispositional mindfulness as having important health implications for high-level athletes. Although the mechanisms underlying the influence of mindfulness on well-being have not been extensively examined in sport, research with non-athletes suggests that emotional awareness and control, along with tolerance of negative emotions, mediate the link between dispositional mindfulness and PWB (MacDonald & Baxter, 2017). Similar mediational models await testing with high-level athletes.

Summary

Spiritual health represents the most mystical and least well understood of the four dimensions of psychosocial health. Although researchers have investigated links between religiousness and indices of emotional and social health, less is known about the role of sport in enhancing and/or degrading spiritual health. The interrelated concepts of flow, peak experience, and mindfulness offer a small window into the spiritual experiences of high-level athletes, but further work remains to establish the mechanisms by which sport influences athletes' spiritual health, as well as how spiritual health effects overall psychosocial health and well-being in high-level athletes.

References

Abbasian, F., Kia, N. S., Mirmohammadkhani, M., Ghahremanfard, F., & Ghods, E. (2016). Self-esteem and spiritual health in cancer patients under chemotherapy in Semnan University of Medical Sciences in 2014. *Health, Spirituality and Medical Ethics, 3*(4), 29–37.

Apstein, S. (2018). *The control pitcher: As free agency looms, will Clayton Kershaw win it all in L.A.?* Retrieved from https://www.si.com/mlb/2018/05/30/clayton-kershaw-los-angeles-dodgers

Baer, R. A., Smith, G. T., Hopkins, J., Krietemeyer, J., & Toney, L. (2006). Using self-report assessment methods to explore facets of mindfulness. *Assessment, 13*(1), 27–45. doi:10.1177/1073191105283504

Banks, R. (1980). Health and the spiritual dimension: Relationships and implications for professional preparation programs. *Journal of School Health, 50*(4), 195–202. doi:10.1111/j.1746-1561.1980.tb07373.x

Bell, N. T., Johnson, S. R., & Petersen, J. C. (2009). Strength of religious faith of athletes and nonathletes at two NCAA Division III institutions. *Sport Journal, 12*(1), 1.

Bruner, M. W., Boardley, I. D., Benson, A. J., Wilson, K. S., Root, Z., Turnnidge, J., … Côté, J. (2018). Disentangling the relations between social identity and prosocial and antisocial behavior in competitive youth sport. *Journal of Youth and Adolescence, 47*(5), 1113–1127. doi:10.1007/s10964-017-0769-2

Burney, N., Osmany, M., & Khan, W. (2017). Spirituality and psychological well-being of young adults. *Indian Journal of Health and Wellbeing, 8*(12), 1481–1484.

Carmody, J., Reed, G., Kristeller, J., & Merriam, P. (2008). Mindfulness, spirituality, and health-related symptoms. *Journal of Psychosomatic Research, 64*(4), 393–403. doi:10.1016/j.jpsychores.2007.06.015

Cathcart, S., McGregor, M., & Groundwater, E. (2014). Mindfulness and flow in elite athletes. *Journal of Clinical Sport Psychology, 8*(2), 119–141. doi:10.1123/jcsp.2014-0018

Cavar, M., Sekulic, E., & Culjak, Z. (2012). Complex interaction of religiousness with other factors in relation to substance use and misuse among female athletes. *Journal of Religion and Health, 51*(2), 381–389. doi:10.1007/s10943-010-9360-9

Chadeayne, A. (2012). Princeton Tigers rally around teammate to cure rare disease. Retrieved from https://swimswam.com/princeton-tigers-rally-around-teammate-to-cure-rare-disease/

Cobb, S. (1976). Social support as a moderator of life stress. *Psychosomatic Medicine, 38*(5), 300–314. doi:10.1097/00006842-197609000-00003

Csikszentmihalyi, M. (1990). *Flow: The psychology of optimal performance.* New York, NY: Harper and Row.

Donatelle, R. J. (2014). *Health: The basics* (11th ed.). London, United Kingdom: Pearson.

Fernandes, H. M., Machado, R. V., Vilaça-Alves, J., Saavedra, F., Aidar, F. J., & Brustad, R. (2014). Social support and sport injury recovery: An overview of empirical findings and practical implications. *Revista de psicología del deporte, 23*(2), 445–449. [English version]

Francois, R. (2018). *Canadians show support to women's Olympic hockey team after loss.* Retrieved from www.victoriabuzz.com/2018/02/silver-for-canadian-womens-hockey/

Galli, N., & Reel, J. J. (2012). "It was hard, but it was good": A qualitative exploration of stress-related growth in Division I intercollegiate athletes. *Qualitative Research in Sport, Exercise and Health, 4*, 297–319. doi:10.1080/2159676X.2012.693524

Gustafsson, H., Davis, P., Skoog, T., Kenttä, G., & Haberl, P. (2015). Mindfulness and its relationship with perceived stress, affect, and burnout in elite junior athletes. *Journal of Clinical Sport Psychology, 9.* doi:10.1123/jcsp.2014-0051.

Hawks, S. (1994). Spiritual health: Definition and theory. *Wellness Perspectives, 10*(4), 3.

Helgeson, V. S. (1993). Two important distinctions in social support: Kind of support and perceived versus received. *Journal of Applied Psychology, 23*(10), 825–845. doi:10.1111/j.1559-1816.1993.tb01008.x

Jackson, S. A. (2008). Athletes in flow: A qualitative investigation of flow states in elite figure skaters. *Journal of Applied Sport Psychology, 4*(2), 161–180. doi:10.1080/10413209208406459

Jafari, M., Ebad, T. S., Rezaei, M., & Ashtarian, H. (2017). Association between spiritual health and depression in students. *Health, Spirituality and Medical Ethics, 4*(2), 12–16.

Jamali, N., Shakerinia, I., Jalili Nikoo, S., & Ghasemi Jobaneh, R. (2017). Role of spiritual health and emotional regulation in mental health of nulliparous women. *Health, Spirituality and Medical Ethics, 4*(3), 32–37.

Johnston, L. H., & Carroll, D. (1998). The provision of social support to injured athletes: A qualitative analysis. *Journal of Sport Rehabilitation, 7*(4), 267–284. doi:10.1123/jsr.7.4.267

Jowett, S. (2017). Coaching effectiveness: The coach–athlete relationship at its heart. *Current Opinion in Psychology, 16*, 154–158. doi:10.1016/j.copsyc.2017.05.006

Jowett, S., & Cockerill, M. (2003). Olympic medallists' perspective of the althlete–coach relationship. *Psychology of Sport and Exercise, 4*(4), 313–331. doi:10.1016/S1469-0292(02)00011-0

Kabat-Zinn, J. (1994). *Wherever you go, there you are: Mindfulness meditation in everyday life.* New York, NY: Hachette Books.

Kaiseler, M., Poolton, J. M., Backhouse, S. H., & Stanger, N. (2017). The relationship between mindfulness and life stress in student-athletes: The mediating role of coping effectiveness and decision rumination. *The Sport Psychologist, 31*(3), 288–298. doi:10.1123/tsp.2016-0083

Keyes, C. L. M. (1998). Social well-being. *Social Psychology Quarterly, 61*(2), 121–140. doi:10.2307/2787065

Koenig, H., Parkerson, G. R., Jr., & Meador, K. G. (1997). Religion index for psychiatric research. *American Journal of Psychiatry, 154*(6), 885–886. doi:10.1176/ajp.154.6.885b

Kumar, S. (2015). Influence of spirituality on burnout and job satisfaction: A study of academic professionals in Oman. *South Asian Journal of Management, 22*(3), 137–175.

Lakey, B. (2010). Social support: Basic research and new strategies for intervention. In J. E. Maddux & J. P. Tangney (Eds.), *Social psychological foundations of clinical psychology* (pp. 177–194). New York, NY: Guilford Press.

Le Bars, H., Gernigon, C., & Ninot, G. (2009). Personal and contextual determinants of elite young athletes' persistence or dropping out over time. *Scandinavian Journal of Medicine & Science in Sports, 19*(2), 274–285. doi:10.1111/j.1600-0838.2008.00786.x

Lee, A. (2011). *The 25 most religious athletes.* Retrieved from https://bleacherreport.com/articles/962060-the-25-most-religious-athletes

Lee, J., & Opio, T. (2011). Coming to America: Challenges and difficulties faced by African student athletes. *Sport, Education and Society, 16*(5), 629–644. doi:10.1080/13 573322.2011.601144

Lundqvist, C., & Sandin, F. (2014). Well-being in elite sport: Dimensions of hedonic and eudaimonic well-being among elite orienteers. *The Sport Psychologist, 28,* 245–254. doi:10.1123/tsp.2013-0024

MacDonald, H. Z., & Baxter, E. E. (2017). *Mindfulness,* 8, 398. Retrieved from https:// doi.org/10.1007/s12671-016-0611-z

Macdougall, H., O'Halloran, P., Sherry, E., & Shields, N. (2016). Needs and strengths of Australian para-athletes: Identifying their subjective psychological, social, and physical health and well-being. *The Sport Psychologist, 30*(1), 1–12. doi:10.1123/ tsp.2015-0006

Marsh, H. W., Perry, C., Horsely, C., & Roche, L. (1995). Multidimensional self-concepts of elite athletes: How do they differ from the general population? *Journal of Sport & Exercise Psychology, 17*(1), 70–83. doi:10.1123/jsep.17.1.70

Moen, F., Abrahamsen, F. A., & Federici, R. A. (2015). Examining possible relationships between mindfulness, stress, school- and sport performances and athlete burnout. *International Journal of Coaching Science, 9*(1), 3–19.

Moore, E. W., Berkley-Patton, J. Y., & Hawes, S. M. (2013). Religiosity, alcohol use, and sex behaviors among college student-athletes. *Journal of Religion and Health, 52*(3), 930–940. doi:10.1007/s10943-011-9543-z

Niwa, T. (1993). The cultural characteristics of sports: Especially concerning the implicit norms of sports as seen in the attitudes of Japanese university athletes. *Japanese Journal of Experimental Social Psychology, 32*(3), 241–258. doi:10.2130/jjesp.32.241

Plante, T. G., Vallaeys, C. L., Sherman, A. C., & Wallston, K. A. (2002). The development of a brief version of the Santa Clara Strength of Religious Faith Questionnaire. *Pastoral Psychology, 50*(5), 359–368. doi:10.1023/A:1014413720710

Ravizza, K. (1977). Peak experiences in sport. *Journal of Humanistic Psychology, 17*(4), 35–40. doi:10.1177/002216787701700404

religion. (2018). In *Merriam-Webster.* Retrieved from https://www.merriam-webster. com/dictionary/religion

Rosenfeld, L. B., Richman, J. M., & Hardy, C. J. (1989). Examining social support networks among athletes: Description and relationship to stress. *The Sport Psychologist, 3*(1), 23–33. doi:10.1123/tsp.3.1.23

Russell, W. D. (2001). An examination of flow state occurrence in college athletes. *Journal of Sport Behavior, 24,* 83–107.

Ryff, C. D. (1989). Happiness is everything, or is it? Explorations on the meaning of psychological well-being. *Journal of Personality and Social Psychology, 57*(6), 1069–1081.

Sheridan, D., Coffee, P., & Lavalee, D. (2014). A systematic review of social support in youth sport. *International Review of Sport and Exercise Psychology, 7*(1), 198–228. doi:10.1080/1750984X.2014.931999

Storch, E. A., & Storch, J. B. (2002a). Correlations for organizational, nonorganizational, and intrinsic religiosity with social support among intercollegiate athletes. *Psychological Reports, 91*(1), 333–334. doi:10.2466/pr0.2002.91.1.333

Storch, E. A., & Storch, J. B. (2002b). Intrinsic religiosity and aggression in a sample of intercollegiate athletes. *Psychological Reports, 91*(3), 1041.

Storch, E. A., Kolsky, A. R., Silvestri, S. M., & Storch, J. B. (2001). Religiosity of elite college athletes. *The Sport Psychologist, 15*(3), 346–351. doi:10.1123/tsp.15.3.346

Storch, E. A., Storch, J. B., & Adams, B. G. (2002). Intrinsic religiosity and social anxiety of intercollegiate athletes. *Psychological Reports, 91*(1), 186. doi:10.2466/ pr0.2002.91.1.186

Storch, E. A., Storch, J. B., Welsh, E., & Okun, A. (2002). Religiosity and depression in intercollegiate athletes. *College Student Journal*, *36*(4), 526.

Storch, E. A., Storch, J. B., Kovacs, A. H., & Okun, A. (2003). Intrinsic religiosity and substance use in intercollegiate athletes. *Journal of Sport & Exercise Psychology*, *25*(2), 248–252. doi:10.1123/jsep.25.2.248

Storch, E. A., Kovacs, A. H., Roberti, J. W., Bailey, L. M., Bravata, E. A., & Storch, J. B. (2004). Strength of religious faith and psychological adjustment in intercollegiate athletes. *Psychological Reports*, *94*(1), 48–50.

Storch, E. A., Roberti, J. W., Heidgerken, A. D., Storch, J. B., Lewin, A. B., Killiany, E. M., … Geffken, G. R. (2004). The Duke Religion Index: A psychometric investigation. *Pastoral Psychology*, *53*(2), 175–181. doi:10.1023/B:PASP.0000046828.94211.53

Stuntz, C. P., & Weiss, M. R. (2009). Achievement goal orientations and motivational outcomes in youth sport: The role of social orientations. *Psychology of Sport and Exercise*, *10*(2), 255–262. Retrieved from https://experts.umn.edu/en/publications/ achievement-goal-orientations-and-motivational-outcomes-in-youth-

Uchino, B. N. (2009). Understanding the links between social support and physical health: A life-span perspective with emphasis on the separability of perceived and received support. *Perspectives on Psychological Science*, *4*(3), 236–255. doi:10.1111/j.1745-6924.2009.01122.x

Udry, E. (1997). Coping and social support among injured athletes following surgery. *Journal of Sport & Exercise Psychology*, *19*(1), 71–90. doi:10.1123/jsep.19.1.71

Wills, T. A. (1991). Social support and interpersonal relationships. In M. S. Clark (Ed.), *Review of personality and social psychology* (Vol. 12, pp. 265–289). Thousand Oaks, CA: Sage.

Wills, T. A., O'Carroll Bantum, E., & Ainette, M. G. (2016). Social support. In Y. Benyamini, M. Johnston, & E. C. Karademas (Eds.), *Assessment in health psychology* (pp. 131-146). Boston, MA: Hogrefe.

World Health Organization. (1998). *Review of the Constitution of the World Health Organization: Report of the Executive Board special group.* Retrieved from apps.who.int/ gb/archive/pdf_files/EB101/pdfangl/angr2.pdf

Wylleman, P. (2000). Interpersonal relationships in sport: Uncharted territory in sport psychology research. *International Journal of Sport Psychology*, *31*, 555–572.

Yaghobi, M., Abdekhoda, M., & Khani, S. (2018). Association between spiritual health and the quality of life in opioid-dependent men in Qom, Iran. *Health, Spirituality and Medical Ethics*, *5*(1), 26–32.

Yang, J., Peek-Asa, C., Lowe, J. B., Heiden, E., & Foster, D. T. (2010). Social support patterns of collegiate athletes before and after injury. *Journal of Athletic Training*, *45*(4), 372–379.

Zenic, N., Stipic, M., & Sekulic, D. (2013). Religiousness as a factor of hesitation against doping behavior in college-age athletes. *Journal of Religion and Health*, *52*(2), 386–396. doi:10.1007/s10943-011-9480-x

PART II

Threats to psychosocial health

High-level athletes' road to success is anything but smooth. In Section II, I address several commonly encountered threats in the sport environment that may not only prevent athletes from achieving their goals but undermine their psychosocial health in the process. *Chapter 4* focuses on the psychosocial health consequences of prolonged exposure to the many environmental, personal, and leadership issues—collectively known as organizational stressors—that athletes must negotiate. In *Chapter 5*, I delve more deeply into one particular organizational stressor- performance pressure, and make a case that an overemphasis on winning and being "the best" is often a major contributor to psychosocial health concerns such as anxiety, depression, substance abuse, and disordered eating.

When winning takes precedence, and coaches, athletes, and sport administrators work as part of a hierarchy of power, athletes are at risk of being emotionally and sexually abused, which is the subject of *Chapter 6*. Within Chapter 6 I discuss the conditions which enable abusive behavior to occur, and the resulting psychosocial health concerns for athletes. Injury is the subject of *Chapter 7*, as I draw from the vast research on psychosocial antecedents and consequences of sport injury. Central nervous system injuries are highlighted as uniquely capable of impacting athletes' emotional, cognitive, and social health. Finally, in *Chapter 8*, I discuss the complexity of transitions for high-level athletes. Whereas in one sense, many transitions are welcomed, and represent the fulfillment of years of work, unexpected transitions can trigger crises. I conclude each chapter with suggestions for advancing knowledge related to that threat.

4

ORGANIZATIONAL STRESS

> Calli is a sophomore playing university lacrosse. After a year of learning as a walk-on, she is excited about the opportunity to compete for a place in the starting lineup and a partial scholarship. Unfortunately things have not gone as she planned. A new coaching staff seems enamored with another player at Calli's same position, and from Calli's perspective, she has been lost in the shuffle. She works hard to get the coaches' attention, but feedback is minimal. Perhaps more important than the playing time itself is the scholarship. Calli currently works on campus part-time in addition to being a full-time student. The scholarship would free her of some of this financial burden. The whole situation has Calli feeling sad, frustrated, and lost.

As Callie's experience suggests, not unlike employees working for a small business or large corporation, when high-level athletes compete as part of a team and/or governing body, conflicts related to organizational functioning, and athletes' place within it, are certain to occur. In fact, in high-level sport, stress associated with aspects of the sport organization may be even more pervasive and wide-reaching than competitive stress (Hanton & Fletcher, 2005). First noted by scholars in industrial-organizational and general psychology, *organizational stress* (aka, occupational stress, job stress, job strain, or workplace stress) refers to any stress related to individuals' job or occupation (Rowney & Cahoon, 1984). Others have adopted a definition rooted in Lazarus' (1966) definition of stress, such that organizational stress refers to a discrepancy between workplace demands and workers' perceived resources (Ongori & Agolla, 2008). When individuals, including athletes, (a) perceive that the demands placed on them by their team or organization pose a threat to their performance and satisfaction, and (b) perceive little control over their situation, distress is likely to occur (Colligan & Higgins, 2006). Karasek's (1979) model of job strain supports the preceding definition, as it posits that *high strain* jobs are those combining high demands with low decision latitude (i.e., autonomy).

Depending on factors such as geography, gender, and the nature of the job, organizational stress can arise from a variety of sources, including frequent in-fighting, excessive workloads, feelings of isolation, role conflict and ambiguity, lack of autonomy, and harassment (Colligan & Higgins, 2006). The latest prevalence estimates suggest that approximately one-third of workers in the U.S. and European Union experience organizational stress, which can result in a variety of deleterious cognitive, emotional, and social health consequences (Colligan & Higgins, 2006; Naghieh, Montgomery, Bonell, Thompson, & Aber, 2015; NIOSH, 1999).

In this chapter, I present an overview of organizational stress as it applies to high-level athletes. First, I briefly discuss the common models used to explain organizational stress that are most relevant to high-level sport. Second, I review research and theory specific to organizational stress in high-level sport. Finally, I discuss the consequences of organizational stress for high-level athletes' psychosocial health.

Psychological models of organizational stress

Although several models of organizational stress have been proposed, the following are those most germane to the high-level sport environment. Consistent with an interactional view of stress and coping, all of the models recognize organizational stress as an interactive process between individuals and their environment.

Person-environment fit model

One of the earliest models of organizational stress was proposed by Pervin (1968), who suggested that incongruence between individuals' personal characteristics and their work environment is the primary cause of stress in the workplace. Person-environment incongruence can occur in one of two ways: (a) a misfit between individuals' knowledge, skills, and abilities, and task requirements, or (b) a misfit between individuals' needs and the resources provided by the organization. Within high-level sport, misfit may occur when a player is frequently asked to perform unlearned skills in high-pressure situations, or when an athlete desires access to specific training equipment that the organization does not have.

Job demands-resources model

In response to other models of organizational stress focused on a limited number of factors that may not be relevant for all occupations, Demerouti, Bakker,

Nachreiner, and Schaufeli (2001) suggested the Job Demands-Resources Model (JD-R) as an alternative. Demerouti et al. posit that organizational stress arises out of an imbalance between the demands of a task (e.g., aspects of the job requiring expenditure of time and effort) and the resources provided to complete the task (e.g., availability of social support, provision choice in decision-making). Stress results when organizational demands exceed organizational resources. Further, resources may buffer the influence of demands, such that the relationship between demands and negative affect is lessened in the presence of resources (Balducci, Schaufeli, & Fraccaroli, 2011). One situation in which the JD-R model may explain organizational stress in high-level sport is when training frequency and duration is high, but financial support is low, causing athletes to work a job in addition to their sport training.

Effort-reward imbalance model

Another more recent model of organizational stress was proposed by Siegrist (1996), who attributed such stress to an imbalance between individuals' perceptions of effort given and rewards received. According to the Effort-Reward Imbalance (ERI) Model, organizational stress will result when (a) effort, manifesting in extrinsic factors such as task demands and intrinsic factors such as a high need for control, are high, and (b) perceptions of rewards in the form of money, esteem, and prospects for advancement, are low. This model seems particularly relevant for high-level sport, in which rewards are readily, and often disproportionately, rewarded. For example, the U.S. women's national soccer team (USWNT), despite playing more games, winning more games (including the 2015 World Cup), and generating more revenue than the U.S. men's national soccer team (USMNT) in 2015, between 2008 and 2015 the top 50 highest paid women were paid one quarter the amount of the top 50 highest paid men (Das, 2016).

Cybernetic theory

The preceding example of pay discrepancy between the USWNT and the USMNT also provides a useful backdrop for the Cybernetic Theory of organizational stress proposed by Edwards (1992). Drawing from the field of cybernetics, which emphasizes systems as functioning through a negative feedback loop, Edwards suggests that organizational stress and associated psychosocial health decrements arise when individuals perceive a discrepancy between their *actual* state within the organization, and their *desired* state. Such a discrepancy may prompt individuals to cope by either changing their desired state or their actual state. In the case of the USWNT, organizational stress was prompted by a discrepancy between their total pay (actual state) to that of the USMNT (desired state). The players coped by filing a complaint of wage discrimination against U.S. Soccer in an attempt to alter their actual state.

Organizational stress in high-level sport

Much of the work on organizational stress in sport has been produced by Fletcher and colleagues (e.g., Fletcher & Hanton, 2003; Hanton & Fletcher, 2005; Didymus & Fletcher, 2017). However, the first investigation of organizational stress in high-level sport was conducted by Woodman and Hardy (2001), who interviewed 16 international-level performers (those with World Championship and/or Olympic Games experience) from the same United Kingdom national team regarding stress caused by their organization. Athletes noted environmental issues related to team selection, finances, training, and travel accommodations, personal issues centering on nutrition, injury, and expectations, leadership issues related to problems with their coach, and team issues in the form of poor communication, role conflict, and an unsatisfactory team atmosphere. The findings were replicated in a similar study by Fletcher and Hanton (2003), thus prompting a call for sport psychology practitioners to recognize and address organizational stress as part of the consulting process, rather than reduce all stress-related issues to the level of individual athletes.

More recently, Lazarus and Folkman's (1984) transactional model of stress and coping has been employed to understand the appraisal and coping of high-level athletes in response to organizational stress. The many and varied sources of organizational stress in the sport environment prompt diverse, and sometimes co-occurring, coping strategies. Not surprisingly, social support seeking is a common strategy used by athletes to manage organizational stressors such as coach issues, demanding travel, and concerns with the competitive environment (Kristiansen & Roberts, 2010; Kristiansen, Murphy, & Roberts, 2012). For example, an athlete experiencing conflict with her coach is likely to seek emotional support in the form of understanding and validation from family and teammates, and coaches themselves are expected to offer informational support in the event of a last-minute scheduling change at a competition. Athletes also rely heavily on *problem-focused* coping strategies (e.g., establishment of a routine, cognitive reframing, effective use of distractions) to modify the circumstances and/or thought processes underlying organizational stress (Kristiansen et al., 2012). Such a head-on approach to coping is often carefully balanced with *avoidance,* in which athletes choose to withdraw from a situation both physically and mentally. Avoidance may be a wise coping strategy, when, for example, an athlete is unhappy with team dynamics, but needs to focus on preparing himself for an upcoming match.

Citing a need to better understand the links between organizational stressors, appraisals, coping, perceived coping effectiveness, and performance satisfaction, Didymus and Fletcher (2017) interviewed ten elite female field hockey players. The players noted numerous organizational stressors, including team culture issues, logistical issues, and personal issues, each of which were defined by one or more situational properties (e.g., degree of ambiguity, novelty, timing, uncertainty). In support of coping with organizational stress as a complex and individual process, several stressors were reported as leading to more than one type of cognitive appraisal across athletes (e.g., dietary stressors were linked to both challenge and threat appraisals), and depending on the athlete, the same coping strategy was reported as either leading to performance satisfaction or performance dissatisfaction.

Taken together, almost two decades of research on organizational stress in high-level athletes reveals some consistency regarding sources of organizational stress (e.g., coaches, team culture, logistical challenges), as well as ways of coping (e.g., social support, problem-focused methods) used by athletes. Didymus and Fletcher (2017) highlight the complexity of the coping process and underscore the importance of appraisals in determining athletes' performance satisfaction. Interestingly, sport researchers have failed to consider common theoretical frameworks of organizational stress when studying the construct in athletes. Furthermore, the psychosocial health implications of organizational stressors for athletes remain unclear. In the following section I rely on both general and sport literature to highlight the implications of organizational stress for athletes' psychosocial health.

Psychosocial health implications of organizational stress for high-level athletes

As with research on stress in general, the physical health consequences of organizational stress are well documented, and include illness (Wang et al., 2014), cardiovascular complications (Theorell & Karasek, 1996), and obesity (Brunner, Chandola, & Marmot, 2007). In terms of psychosocial health, organizational stress has been linked to an increased risk for a variety of depressive disorders in the general population (e.g., Burns, Butterworth, & Antsey, 2016; Wang, Schmitz, Dewa, & Stansfeld, 2009). A meta-analysis of 11 studies conducted between 1994 and 2005 showed associations between elements of organizational stress (e.g., high demands with low autonomy, high effort with low rewards) and common psychological disorders (Stansfeld & Candy, 2006). Recognizing organizational stress as a threat to worker health and well-being, researchers at the National Institute for Occupational Safety and Health (NIOSH; 1999) proposed a theoretical model of job stress and health to guide further research and practice (Hurrell & Sauter, 2012). In the model, the researchers posit that work stress in the form of task demands, organizational factors, and physical conditions, and as moderated by individual, non-work, and buffer factors such as social support, lead to acute psychological (e.g., changes in affect), physiological (e.g., cardiovascular complications), and behavioral (e.g., changes in sleep) reactions, which can over time result in cardiovascular disease, clinical psychological disorders, and/or long-term physical impairment (Hurrell & Sauter, 2012).

Of interest for the current text are the psychological and behavioral consequences of organizational stress. Although the NIOSH model has not been employed when studying high-level athletes, it offers a useful framework for doing so. When considered in the context of extant research on organizational stress in high-level athletes, the model can easily be modified to guide research and practice with this population. For example, imagine an elite track athlete who competes for her country's national team. Research on organizational stress in athletes suggests that this athlete may experience organizational stress in the form of financial constraints, team selection, conflict with coaches, and/or issues related to team cohesion. Perhaps she comes from an unstable family environment and has insufficient tools with which to cope with the organizational stressors. The combination of high organizational stress and difficult non-sport circumstances may in turn lead to feelings of depression and perhaps the adoption of unhealthy behaviors such as excessive alcohol consumption and/or poor sleep hygiene. Without intervention, she risks long-term psychosocial health consequences such as clinical depression, substance dependence, and social isolation.

The previous scenario suggests how the process of organizational stress from onset to long-term outcome may occur for high-level athletes. However, a notable absence from the NIOSH model is the underlying mechanisms by which organizational stress leads to adverse psychosocial health outcomes. Diminished self-esteem and low perceived mastery over the working environment are two psychological constructs implicated as mediating the relationship between work stress and negative emotional health outcomes in non-athletes (Cole, Ibrahim, Shannon, Scott, & Eyles, 2002). Conceptually, perceived mastery over one's environment is much like Ryan and Deci's (1999) notion of *autonomy*, or individuals' need for personal choice in a given situation. Autonomy is, along with competence and relatedness, one of three basic psychosocial needs identified by Deci and Ryan in their self-determination theory (SDT) of motivation. Based on a eudaimonic approach to human motivation and well-being, SDT postulates that satisfaction of the three needs promotes motivation grounded in the intrinsic values of learning, stimulation, and accomplishment (Deci & Ryan, 2000; Ryan, Huta, & Deci, 2013). Although basic psychosocial need satisfaction is important for motivation, the needs are, in and of themselves, indicators of well-being (Deci & Ryan, 2000).

Guided by principles of SDT and Lazarus and Folkman's (1984) transactional model of stress and coping, Bartholomew, Arnold, Hampson, and Fletcher (2017) examined the links between organizational stressors, cognitive appraisals, and need satisfaction/thwarting in over 300 high-level British athletes from a variety of sports. The researchers found that when athletes perceived the frequency and intensity of organizational stressors as posing a threat to their future well-being (i.e., threat appraisal), they were more likely to report psychosocial need frustration (e.g., feeling overly controlled, feeling rejected). By contrast, when athletes appraised the duration of organizational stressors as an opportunity for growth (i.e., challenge appraisal), they were more likely to experience need satisfaction. Moreover, challenge appraisals predicted perceptions of control over the stressor, which in turn positively predicted need satisfaction and negatively predicted need frustration. Appraisals of threat predicted perceived lack of control, and subsequent need frustration. These findings support the notion that athletes' perceptions of stressors in the sport environment play an important role in determining the effect of these stressors on psychosocial health.

Another adverse psychosocial health outcome that may be linked to organizational stress in high-level sport, is burnout. As originally defined by Maslach and Jackson (1984), and later adapted for sport by Raedeke (1997), *burnout* refers to "a syndrome of physical/emotional exhaustion, sport devaluation, and reduced athletic accomplishment among athletes" (p. 398). Originally observed and studied in professionals who worked in helping professions, not only is burnout a concerning phenomenon in its own right, but also because of links with heart disease (Toker, Melamed, Berliner, Zeltser, & Shapira, 2012), depression (Bianchia, Schonfeld, & Laurent, 2015), and poorer cognitive health (Sandstrom, Rhodin, Lundberg, Olsson, & Nyberg, 2005).

Within sport, perceived stress has emerged as the most consistent predictor of athlete burnout (Eklund & DeFreese, 2015; Goodger, Gorely, Lavallee, & Harwood, 2007), and Smith's (1986) cognitive-affective model emphasizes the role of chronic stress in contributing to physiological and behavioral outcomes associated with burnout. Tabei, Fletcher, and Goodger (2012) argued that, in addition to personal stress, explanations for burnout should account for the role of organizational stressors. Coakley (1992) was the first to propose that high-level adolescent athletes burn out not only because they lack the personal resources to cope with stress, but because of a sport structure that robs athletes of personal control and makes excessive time demands which prohibit them from expanding their identity beyond sport.

Partially guided by Coakley's (1992) Unidimensional Identity and External Control Model of burnout, Tabei (et al.) undertook a mixed-methods investigation of organizational stress and burnout in 98 English and Japanese university soccer players. Following completion of Raedeke and Smith's (2001) Athlete Burnout Questionnaire, the authors interviewed nine athletes who scored above the threshold for burnout for all three dimensions (i.e., physical and emotional exhaustion, sport devaluation, and reduced sense of accomplishment) for their perceptions on the link between organizational stressors and dimensions of burnout. Ten types of organizational stressors were identified by the players as contributing to at least one dimension of burnout each. For example, the stressor training and competition load (e.g., hard training, insufficient rest) was mentioned by players as contributing to both sport devaluation and physical and emotional exhaustion. In addition, leadership style (e.g., authoritarian coaching style, insufficient coach knowledge) was reported by players as influencing all three dimensions of burnout.

Of further interest was the higher prevalence of burnout in the Japanese players, which, partially based on the follow-up interviews, the authors attributed to the common practice of especially harsh physical conditioning prescribed by Japanese coaches. An emphasis on a hierarchical structure within Japanese sport, in which more junior players are often ignored, and even abused by more experienced players, also seemed to be a factor differentiating the Japanese from the English players. In sum, the lone study of organizational stress and burnout showed that these athletes perceived a link between aspects of their sporting environment and feelings of exhaustion, sport devaluation, and a reduced sense of accomplishment. Unfortunately, researchers have yet to follow up on this study to gain a further understanding of the psychosocial health consequences of organizational stress. In the following section, I offer some possibilities for expanding this line of research.

Future research directions for organizational stress and athlete psychosocial health

At this point, common sources of organizational stress in high-level sport, and subsequent coping process adopted by athletes, are quite well known. Lagging far behind is an understanding of the cognitive, emotional, social, and spiritual health consequences of organizational stress in this population. Although the aforementioned study by Tabei et al. (2012) established organizational stressors as a factor in one psychosocial health outcome of interest, namely burnout, other possible outcomes remain unexplored. For example, as has been found in non-athletes (e.g., Burns et al., 2016) it seems possible that prolonged organizational stress may trigger common psychological disorders such as anxiety, depression, substance abuse, and eating disorders. And given that teammates and coaches are often considered as elements of organizational stress, it behooves researchers to consider the social health ramifications, perhaps via measures of social adjustment (e.g., Weissman & Bothwell, 1976).

Regardless of the chosen outcome, a longitudinal and multivariate approach should be adopted to account for the dynamic nature of organizational stress. Such an approach will allow researchers to understand whether organizational stress does indeed predict future adverse psychosocial outcomes, the relative influence of different sources of organizational stress, and the role of stressor frequency, duration, and intensity (Arnold & Fletcher, 2012). It may also be interesting to examine the transient versus persistent nature of any such outcomes. That is, under what circumstances does stress from the sport environment lead to psychosocial consequences from which athletes recover in a relatively brief time period, rather than a more chronic condition? The answers to such questions will inform attempts to minimize potentially harmful and unnecessary organizational stress, and/or arm athletes with tools to effectively cope.

Perhaps because the majority of organizational stress in sport research has occurred in the United Kingdom, there is a gap in knowledge regarding the nature of organizational stress for American student-athletes competing at NCAA-sponsored institutions. The NCAA has come under scrutiny for failing to fairly compensate student-athletes, and particularly those who play American football and men's basketball at major universities, who spend upwards of 20 hours per week on their sport, and whose $23,000 average annual scholarship represent just a fraction of their estimated value on the open market (Huma & Staurowsky, 2012). Recent efforts by current NCAA athletes to unionize, and by former athletes to sue the NCAA over the unauthorized use of their names and images in merchandise and video games underscore the level of discontent by these individuals (Farrey, 2015; Ganim, 2014). Huma and Staurowsky offer several reasons why student-athletes may experience organizational stress, including (a) denial of athletes to independently profit on their own image, (b) restricting compensation, (c) failing to provide health insurance, (d) placing extreme demands on time and energy, and (e) limiting access to due process. Based on the aforementioned conditions, research examining perceptions of organizational stress and psychosocial health of collegiate American football and men's basketball players at major universities seems warranted.

Conclusion

The world of high-level sport, while often viewed as glamorous and highly desirable, is also fraught with challenges related to issues of relationships, finances, and selection procedures. When stressors exceed athletes' resources, psychosocial health may be adversely affected. Although researchers have done well to identify the most common organizational stressors for high-level athletes, as well as the common coping strategies employed, less is known about the long-term psychosocial consequences. Moving forward, models used to understand organizational stress in non-sport settings should be tested with high-level athletes. In addition to further exploration of the link between organizational stressors and burnout, there is a need for longitudinal studies tracking various indices of psychosocial health, with an emphasis on the emotional and social implications. Finally, based on inequities in compensation and overly restrictive conditions, there is a need to examine the link between organizational stress and psychosocial health in football and men's basketball players at major revenue-producing NCAA athletics programs.

References

Arnold, R., & Fletcher, D. (2012). A research synthesis and taxonomic classification of the organizational stressors encountered by sport performers. *Journal of Sport & Exercise Psychology*, *34*(3), 397–429. doi:10.1123/jsep.34.3.397

Balducci, C., Fraccaroli, F., & Schaufeli, W. B. (2011). The job demands–resources model and counterproductive work behaviour: The role of job-related affect. *European Journal of Work and Organizational Psychology*, *20*(4), 467–496. doi:10.1080/1061580 6.2011.555533

Bianchia, R., Schonfeld, S. I., & Laurent, E. (2015). Burnout–depression overlap: A review. *Clinical Psychology Review*, *36*, 28–41. doi:10.1016/j.cpr.2015.01.004

Bartholomew, K. J., Arnold, R., Hampson, R. J., & Fletcher, D. (2017). Organizational stressors and basic psychological needs: The mediating role of athletes' appraisal mechanisms. *Scandinavian Journal of Medicine & Science in Sports*, *27*, 2127–2139. doi:10.1111/sms.12851

Brunner, E. J., Chandola, T., & Marmot, M. G. (2007). Prospective effect of job strain on general and central obesity in the Whitehall II Study. *American Journal of Epidemiology*, *165*(7), 828–837. doi:10.1093/aje/kwk058

Burns, R. A., Butterworth, P., & Anstey, K. J. (2016). An examination of the long-term impact of job strain on mental health and wellbeing over a 12-year period. *Social Psychiatry and Psychiatric Epidemiology*, *51*. 725–733. doi:10.1007/s00127-016-1192-9

Coakley, J. (1992). Burnout among adolescent athletes: A personal failure or social problem? [Presidential Address.] *Sociology of Sport Journal*, *9*(3), 271–285. doi:10.1123/ssj.9.3.271

Cole, D. C., Ibrahim, S., Shannon, H. S., Scott, F. E., & Eyles, J. (2002). Work and life stressors and psychological distress in the Canadian working population: A structural equation modelling approach to analysis of the 1994 National Population Health Survey. *Journal of Chronic Diseases in Canada*, *23*(3), 91–99.

Colligan, T. W., & Higgins, E. M. (2006). Workplace stress: Etiology and consequences. *Journal of Workplace Behavioral Health*, *21*(2), 89–97. doi:10.1300/J490v21n02_07

Das, A. (2016, March 31). Top female players accuse U.S. soccer of wage discrimination. *The New York Times*. Retrieved from https://www.nytimes.com/2016/04/01/sports/soccer/uswnt-us-women-carli-lloyd-alex-morgan-hope-solo-complain.html

Deci, E. L., & Ryan, R. M. (1985). *Intrinsic motivation and self-determination in human behavior*. New York, NY: Plenum Press.

Demerouti, E., Bakker, A. B., Nachreiner, F. S., & Wilmar, B. (2001). The job demands–resources model of burnout. *Journal of Applied Psychology*, *86*(3), 499–512.

Didymus, F. F., & Fletcher, D. (2017). Effects of a cognitive–behavioral intervention on field hockey players' appraisals of organizational stressors. *Psychology of Sport and Exercise*, *30*, 173–185. doi:10.1016/j.psychsport.2017.03.005

Edwards, J. R. (1992). A cybernetic theory of stress, coping, and well-being in organizations. *Academy of Management Review*, *17*, No. 2. doi:10.5465/amr.1992.4279536

Eklund, R., & DeFreese, J. D. (2015). Athlete burnout: What we know, what we could know, and how we can find out more. *International Journal of Applied Sports Sciences*, *27*(2), 63–75.

Farrey, T. (2015, August 17). *Northwestern players denied request to form first union for athletes*. Retrieved from http://www.espn.com/college-football/story/_/id/13455477/nlrb-says-northwestern-players-cannot-unionize

Fletcher, D., & Hanton, S. (2003). Sources of organizational stress in elite sports performers. *The Sport Psychologist*, *17*(2). 175–195. doi:10.1123/tsp.17.2.175

Ganim, S. (2014, June 19). Paying college athletes would hurt traditions, NCAA chief Emmert testifies. *CNN*. Retrieved from https://www.cnn.com/2014/06/19/us/ncaa-obannon-lawsuit-trial/index.html

Goodger, K., Gorely, T., Lavallee, D., & Harwood, C. (2007). Burnout in sport: A systematic review. *The Sport Psychologist*, *21*(2), 127–151. doi:10.1123/tsp.21.2.127

Hanton, S., & Fletcher, D. (2005). Organizational stress in competitive sport: More than we bargained for? *International Journal of Sport Psychology*, *36*(4), 273–283.

Huma, R., & Staurowsky, E. J. (2012). *The $6 billion heist: Robbing college athletes under the guise of amateurism*. Retrieved from https://www.ncpanow.org/six-billion-heist

Hurrell, J. J., Jr., & Sauter, S. L. (2012). Occupational stress: Causes, consequences, prevention, and intervention. In A. M. Rossi, P. L. Perrewe, & J. A. Meurs (Eds.), *Coping and prevention* (pp. 231-248. Charlotte, NC: Information Age.

Karasek, R. A. (1979). Job demands, job decision latitude, and mental strain: Implications for job redesign. *Administrative Science Quarterly*, *24*, 285–308. doi:10.2307/2392498

Kristiansen, E., Murphy, D., & Roberts, G. C. (2012). Organizational stress and coping in U.S. professional soccer. *Journal of Applied Sport Psychology*, *24*(2), 207–223. doi:10.1080/10413200.2011.614319

Kristiansen, E., & Roberts, G. C. (2010). Young elite athletes and social support: Coping with competitive and organizational stress in "Olympic" competition. *Scandinavian Journal of Medicine and Science in Sports*, *20*(4), 686–695. doi:10.1111/j.1600-0838.2009.00950.x

Lazarus, R. S. (1966). *Psychological stress and the coping process.* New York, NY: McGraw-Hill.

Lazarus, R. S., & Folkman, S. (1984). Coping and adaptation. In W. D. Gentry (Ed.), *The handbook of behavioral medicine* (pp. 282–325). New York, NY: Guilford.

Maslach, C., & Jackson, S. E. (1984). Burnout in organizational settings. *Applied Social Psychology Annual*, *5*, 133–153.

Naghieh, A., Montgomery, P., Bonell, C. P., Thompson, M., & Aber, J. L. (2015). Organisational interventions for improving wellbeing and reducing work-related stress in teachers. *Cochrane Database of Systematic Reviews*, *8*(4), CD010306. doi:10.1002/14651858.CD010306.pub2

National Institute for Occupational Safety and Health. (1999). *Stress ... at work* (DHHS [NIOSH] Publication Number 99-101). Retrieved from https://www.cdc.gov/niosh/docs/99-101/default.html

Ongori, H., & Agolla, J. E. (2008). Occupational stress in organizations and its effects on organizational performance. *Journal of Management Research*, *8*(3), 123–135.

Pervin, L. A. (1968). Performance and satisfaction as a function of individual–environment fit. *Psychological Bulletin*, *69*(1), 56–68. doi:10.1037/h0025271

Raedeke, T. D. (1997). Is athlete burnout more than just stress? A sport commitment perspective. *Journal of Sport and Exercise Psychology*, *19*(4), 396–417. doi:10.1123/jsep.19.4.396

Raedeke, T. D., & Smith, A. L. (2001). Development and preliminary validation of an athlete burnout measure. *Journal of Sport & Exercise Psychology*, *23*(4), 281–306. doi:10.1123/jsep.23.4.281

Rowney, J. L., & Cahoon, A. R. (1984). The challenge of organizational stress. *Organization Development Journal*, *2*(2), 25–32.

Ryan, R. M., & Deci, E. L. (1999). Intrinsic and extrinsic motivations: Classic definitions and new directions. *Contemporary Educational Psychology*, *25*(1), 54–67. doi:10.1006/ceps.1999.1020

Ryan, R. M., Huta, V., & Deci, E. L. (2013). Living well: A self-determination theory perspective on eudaimonia. *Journal of Happiness Studies*, *9*, 139–170. doi:10.1007/978-94-007-5702-8_7

Sandström, A., Rhodin, I. N., Lundberg, M., & Olssona, R., & Nyberg, L. (2005). Impaired cognitive performance in patients with chronic burnout syndrome. *Biological Psychology*, *69*(3), 271–279. doi:10.1016/j.biopsycho.2004.08.003

Siegrist, J. (1996). Adverse health effects of high-effort/low-reward conditions. *Journal of Occupational Health Psychology*, *1*(1), 27–41.

Stansfeld, S., & Candy, B. (2006). Psychosocial work environment and mental health—A meta-analytic review. *Scandinavian Journal of Work, Environment & Health*, *32*(6), 443–462. Retrieved from http://www.jstor.org/stable/40967597

Tabei, Y., Fletcher, D., & Goodger, K. (2012). The relationship between organizational stressors and athlete burnout in soccer players. *Journal of Clinical Sport Psychology*, *6*(2), 146–165. doi:10.1123/jcsp.6.2.146

Theorell, T., & Karasek, R. A. (1996). Current issues relating to psychosocial job strain and cardiovascular disease research. *Journal of Occupational Health Psychology*, *1*(1), 9–26.

Toker, S., Melamed, S., Berliner, S., Zeltser, D., & Shapira, I. (2012). Burnout and risk of coronary heart disease: A prospective study of 8838 employees. *Psychosomatic Medicine*, *74*(8), 840–847. doi:10.1097/PSY.0b013e31826c3174

Wang, J. L., Schmitz, N., Dewa, C., & Stansfeld, S. (2009). Changes in perceived job strain and the risk of major depression: Results from a population-based longitudinal study. *American Journal of Epidemiology*, *169*(9), 1085–1091. doi:10.1093/aje/kwp037

Wang, M. J., Mykletun, A., Møyner, E. I., Øverland, S., Henderson, M., Stansfeld, S., … Harvey, S. B. (2014). Job strain, health and sickness absence: Results from the Hordaland Health Study. *PLOS ONE*, *9*(4), e96025. doi:10.1371/journal.pone.0096025

Weissman, M. M., & Bothwell, S. (1976). Assessment of social adjustment by patient self-report. *Archives of General Psychiatry*, *33*(9), 1111–1115. doi:10.1001/archpsyc.1976.01770090101010

Woodman, T., & Hardy, L. (2001). A case study of organizational stress in elite sport. *Journal of Applied Sport Psychology*, *13*(2), 207–238. doi:10.1080/104132001753149892

5

PERFORMANCE PRESSURE

Emery is a top performer for a professional rugby team. Beginning with development camps as a five-year-old, he has dedicated nearly his entire 25 years to the sport through year-round training. Over the years, his parents and coaches have been a constant source of motivation, as they push him to be the best that he can be. Every major life decision he has made has on some level involved consideration of rugby. Although he has been told that occasional breaks from the sport are important for his recovery and overall well-being, Emery finds it difficult to "slack off." Recent success at the professional level has raised his profile both locally and nationally, and considerably increased his responsibilities to sponsors and media. It seems that he cannot escape the media's attention, as they somehow manage to be wherever he is with a camera and questions. Tasked with meeting these new demands along with maintaining a high level of performance, Emery has been feeling "off" for the last several months. His motivation for rugby, usually never in question, has waned, and he is seemingly always mentally and physically exhausted. No longer able to push through, Emery abruptly dropped out of an Australian tour, citing a stomach illness.

Inherent to life as a high-level athlete is the expectation of consistently strong performance across varied competitive situations, while simultaneously maintaining a balanced life and serving as a positive role model. As former USMNT soccer player Landon Donovan said in a 2013 interview, "I think we have this perception that people who are athletes or celebrities are not susceptible to the same problems as everyone else. There's a lot of travel, there's a lot of demands, there's a lot of *pressure* [emphasis added]—both internal and external" (HuffPost, para. 2).

As noted by Donovan, and illustrated in the hypothetical example of Emery, the lifestyle of high-level athletics, while seemingly glamorous, can also prove taxing due to demands from themselves and others.

Within high-level sport, the notion of *psychological pressure* is often used reductively to connote specific competitive situations in which athletes' immediate performance determines success or failure in a high-stakes evaluative setting. Such pressure is often studied in conjunction with the notion of choking (e.g., Hill, Carvell, Matthews, Weston, & Thelwell, 2017) or clutch performance (Swann, Crust, Jackman, Vella, Allen, & Keegan, 2017). However, in this chapter I refer to psychological pressure more broadly, as athletes' perceptions of chronic and pervasive demands placed upon them that are either directly or indirectly related to sport performance. These demands may be self-imposed, but often arise due to sport sub-cultures that adopt winning as the primary objective. For example, an international-level figure skater might feel pressure to lose weight in order to: (a) project a more pleasing appearance to her coach and potential judges, and/or (b) allow her to jump higher and move faster, thereby enhancing her scoring potential. The previous example illustrates the multi-faceted nature of pressure, as it emanates from multiple sources (e.g., coach, judges, self), and prompts action toward separate, but related goals (e.g., appearance and performance).

In this chapter I draw from both psychological and sociological literature to discuss the nature of psychological pressure for high-level athletes in various competitive settings, as well as the psychosocial health implications of excessive pressure. I conclude by offering suggestions for further scholarly inquiry in this area.

Winning: The common denominator in psychological pressure

As has been mentioned several times already in this text, most threats to high-level athletes' psychosocial health can ultimately be linked to a strong and often insatiable desire on the part of coaches and other representatives of high-level sport organizations to be "the best." And although the quest for success is not inherently detrimental to athletes' psychosocial health, when not counterbalanced with a focus on holistic athlete development and effective coping skills, athlete health and well-being may be compromised. Sport sociologists have long warned of the potential dangers of an overemphasis on winning in elite sport at both the youth and adult levels. In an early sociological investigation of the win-at-all-cost attitude associated with high-level sport, all-star minor league ice hockey players had a keen awareness of the high expectations for performance set by coaches (Vaz, 1974). One player said, "You're always expected to be the best. No matter what" (p. 48).

In the early 1990s, Coakley brought the issue of a performance-focus to the forefront in papers on burnout in youth sport (1992) and positive deviance in high-level athletes (Hughes & Coakley, 1991). Coakley's empowerment model of burnout is covered in Chapter 4 as it relates to organizational stress, but the model also illustrates how a win–first and performance-focused culture is at the core of burnout in young elite athletes. In short, when winning is the foremost goal of high-level youth sport, athletes' identity may be constricted, and autonomy minimized. The result may be burnout, or, for athletes who do continue, sport may become a detriment rather than an enhancer of psychosocial health and well-being. It should be noted that Coakley conducted the interviews leading to his model in the early 1980s, and it can be argued that elite youth sport has since begun to even further mirror elite collegiate and professional sport, with private travel teams and year-round competition commonplace in sports such as basketball, baseball, soccer, and volleyball. Indeed, current high-level athletes are cognizant of the fact that their non-sport identities are often compromised in the pursuit of sport goals (Hickey & Kelly, 2008).

Around the same time that Coakley proposed his empowerment model of burnout, he and Hughes (1991) critiqued implicit and explicit norms of high-level sport which touts, above all else, values such as sacrificing for the game, striving to get bigger, faster, and stronger, playing through pain and injury, and the belief that anything is possible if one works hard enough. The authors emphasized how the uncritical acceptance of such norms can lead to a variety of deviant and unhealthy behaviors such as performance-enhancing substance abuse, overtraining, and hazing. Research conducted with high-level athletes since 1991 supports athletes' acceptance of performance-focused norms as a normal and natural part of their existence (e.g., Coker-Cranney, Watson, Bernstein, Voelker, & Coakley, 2018), an impetus for doping (e.g., Ohl, Fincouer, Lentillon-Kaestner, Defrance, & Brissoneau, 2015), and a risk factor for injury (e.g., Wiese-Bjornstal, 2000; see Chapter 7 for further details). Also concerning is athletes' willingness to compete while hurt, due to pressure from those in the sport environment that can be either direct (e.g., explicit comments encouraging athletes to perform while hurt) or indirect (e.g., athletes' perceptions of what others will think of they don't play while hurt) (Mayer & Thiel, 2018).

Perhaps the most striking example of the pressure faced by athletes to be the best was Michael Messner's study of sports and masculinity in 30 former high-level male athletes. The interviews revealed the integral link between masculinity and sport success for the men in this study, and how sport was used as a vehicle for men to affirm their sense of masculinity by pushing through pain, abusing drugs, and subjugating women and others in positions of lesser power (Messner, 1995). Particularly for athletes from lower social classes, sport success was symbolic of hyper-masculinity, a source of self-worth, and a way to earn respect from others. One quote from a former football player in Messner's study is emblematic of athletes' beliefs about the link between on-field success and self-identity: "if you weren't on the upside, you were nothing—nobody cared—you were nothing, you had no substance to you, you were a loser" (p. 47). Although overconformity to a power and performance view of sport is most often associated with male athletes, female athletes are certainly not immune, and may themselves succumb to the pressure to experiment with performance-enhancing substances and engage in unhealthy dietary practices in the quest for optimal performance (Waldron & Krane, 2005).

In summary, sociological analyses of sport aid our understanding of the culture underlying psychological pressure for high-level athletes. Specifically, sport sociologists argue that as winning takes precedent, athletes' identity becomes constricted, their lives overly controlled, and the pressure to do whatever it takes to win is enhanced. Such pressure may lead to a less-than-optimal sport experience for athletes, burnout, and harmful behaviors aimed at themselves and others.

The context for psychological pressure in high-level sport

Although an emphasis on winning is similar across all high-level sport environments, the nature of psychological pressure is also dependent on the context in which athletes operate. Two of the most salient factors are competitive level and sport type. I begin with an overview of the similarities and differences in pressure across competitive levels, before addressing the unique pressures encountered by athletes in leanness-focused sports.

The evolution of psychological pressure across competitive levels

From elite youth club teams to professional organizations, athletes are compelled to behave and perform in accordance with the expectations of individuals who exert the most power at that point in time. For high-level youth athletes, parents and coaches are the power-brokers. Youth athletes feel parental pressure whenever parents take ownership of their sport experience, verbally berate athletes about their performance, or worse, shout instructions or feedback during competitions (McCarthy & Jones, 2007). Further, parents can unknowingly exert pressure on their children by committing large amounts of money to support sport participation (Dunn, Dorsch, King, & Rothlisberger, 2016). Paradoxically, despite most overinvolved parents' goal of enhancing their young athletes' sport experience, the resulting pressure more often leads to diminished performance, enjoyment, and commitment (Gould, Lauer, Rolo, Jannes, & Pennisi, 2006; Sánchez-Miguel, Leo, Sánchez-Olivia, Amado, & García-Calvo, 2013). Indeed, the careers and lives of several talented young athletes have been derailed by parents who are more invested in their children's sport performance than the children themselves. Former National Football League quarterback Todd Marinovich and former professional tennis players Andre Agassi and Jennifer Capriati are just a few prominent athletes who faced excessive pressure from their parents at a young age, and encountered personal problems later in life because of it.

Although much less work has been conducted on coach-created psychological pressure in high-level youth sport, there is reason to believe that coaches play a similar role to parents. Most recent studies of youth sport have employed

[margin handwritten note:] over-involved parents

Deci and Ryan's (1985) Self Determination Theory to illustrate coach behaviors that enhance athlete motivation to conclude that young athletes are optimally motivated when coaches exhibit autonomy-supportive behaviors such as inviting input from players on team decisions (e.g., Amorose & Anderson-Butcher, 2015; Jöesaar, Hein, & Hagger, 2012). Because autonomy involves granting athletes personal agency over their sport experience, it can be viewed as the antithesis of psychological pressure (Deci & Ryan, 1985; Stebbings, Taylor, Spray, & Ntoumanis, 2012). Autonomy-supportive behaviors are especially powerful when employed by both the coach and at least one parent (Amorose, Anderson-Butcher, Newman, Fraina, & Iachini, 2016). Coaches who adopt a more controlling style may choose to motivate and/or apply pressure on young athletes using the threat of punishment. Battaglia, Kerr, and Stirling (2017) interviewed competitive youth ice hockey players to understand players' perceptions of punitive strategies used by their coach. All 12 players in the study reported that they had been punished by their coach in the past, and that such punishment took the form of yelling, exercise, cleaning of equipment, and/or benching. Punitive strategies were generally viewed by athletes as having a negative influence on their self-image, relationships, and motivation in sport. Thus, just as with parents, coaches' well-meaning attempts to coax better performance out of young athletes through pressure-inducing strategies such as shouting, shaming, and punishing, can have the opposite of the intended effect.

As athletes advance to the collegiate setting, the source and nature of psychological pressure shifts. While parents become more peripheral, coaches take on a more prominent role, and athletes must learn to balance their academic responsibilities with rigorous practice and competition schedules. Tightly controlled athletics programs restrict athletes' sense of autonomy, and can force athletes to choose between succeeding academically or athletically (Kimball & Freysinger, 2003; Rothschild-Checroune, Gravelle, Dawson, & Karlis, 2012). The presence of scholarships can add further pressure for athletes as they strive to retain financial assistance from year to year (Cooper & Cooper, 2015). Black collegiate athletes in one study noted how the degree of coach control over scholarships more closely resembled a high-powered business arrangement rather than an educational experience (Cooper & Cooper). Although athletes in revenue-producing sports such as football and men's basketball are often the focus of media attention on the problems and pressures faced by college athletes, athletes in non-revenue-producing sports also note time pressure related to balancing academics and athletics (Paule & Gilson, 2010). Indeed, collegiate athletes are in the unenviable position of serving "two masters" when they must comply with the oft-opposing agendas of university instructors and university coaches (Rhatigan, 1984). On one hand, coaches' jobs are often dependent on athletes' on-field success, which may cause them to implicitly or explicitly send the message to athletes that, so long as they remain eligible to play, the team takes priority over the grade. On the other hand, at least in theory, instructors have the same standards of class performance for both athletes and non-athletes. In some cases, instructors possess negative views or stereotypes about athletes and are reluctant to make accommodations for athletes' sport schedule (Parsons, 2013). In such cases, collegiate athletes may feel additional pressure to prove themselves to their instructors.

To summarize, the dynamics of psychological pressure for athletes change at the collegiate level. As parents play a lesser role, coaches exert more control. Athletes must learn to balance the sometimes contradictory demands of coaches and instructors, and work to "win over" instructors who hold negative views of athletes. Finally, it should be noted that most studies reflect the experience of collegiate athletes in the U.S. only, and may not generalize to other countries where government-sponsored athlete-development programs are prominent.

At the international and professional levels of competition, psychological pressure to perform is amplified by financial considerations and increased media attention. Success at the highest level of competition only increases expectations, and for athletes who are not prepared to handle the added pressure associated with being one of the best and most recognizable at what they do, adverse outcomes can occur. One recent example is mixed martial artist Jon Jones, whose rapid ascent to the top of the Ultimate Fighting Championship (UFC) light heavyweight division between 2008 and 2011 made him one of the sport's biggest stars. Unfortunately, a hit-and-run incident in 2015 and multiple doping violations between 2016 and 2017 derailed his career. UFC commissioner Dana White expressed his opinion on the reason for Jones' fall from grace in a 2017 interview:

> Jon Jones came in and just started making millions of dollars immediately and he was, like, 24 years old. And you can go back to interviews of me saying, "That's great, he's talented enough to win the belt. Can he handle the pressure and all the stuff that goes along with being a world champion? With being rich?" And that question got answered.
>
> *(Harkness, 2017, para. 4)*

Although not all stories of struggles with pressure are as pronounced as Jones', athletes competing at the highest levels of their sport must learn to cope with the associated pressure. Of course, fame and fortune are not an issue for all elite athletes. For those who compete in sports that are less mainstream, pressure arises from more traditional sources such as others' expectations, institutional criteria, and self-imposed expectations (McKay, Niven, Lavallee, & White, 2008).

Summary

Although psychological pressure is apparent across all strata of high-level sport, certain sources of pressure are clearly more influential at different times in athletes' careers. For elite youth sport participants, parental and coach pressure is at the forefront, as these individuals often adopt the role of taskmaster for young athletes. At the collegiate level, coaches supersede parents as a source of pressure, and student–athletes are often torn between devoting efforts to their academic and athletic endeavors. And at the highest levels of sport, in addition to pressure from coaches and institutional standards, some athletes in high-profile sports must learn to cope with the pressure of being a celebrity, including increased media scrutiny.

Weight and body pressure for athletes in leanness-focused sports

Although psychological pressure to perform is universal across all high-level sports, certain sports warrant special consideration due to the strong link between body shape and/or body weight and motor performance. As in the previous example of the figure skater, athletes competing in aesthetic (e.g., gymnastics, diving), weight-class (e.g., wrestling, rowing), and endurance (e.g., running, skiing, cycling) sports commonly encounter pressure from coaches, teammates, family, and others to modify their body for maximum performance (Voelker & Galli, in press). In timed sports such as swimming, an overemphasis on main-taining low body weight for enhanced speed can create weight-loss pressure from coaches and others (Reel & Gill, 2001). The skimpy and form-fitting uni-forms worn in sports such as gymnastics, figure skating, diving, and wrestling are an additional source of pressure for both male and female athletes (Galli & Reel, 2009; Voelker & Reel, 2015). Some athletes may also perceive pressure to portray the "look" of a high-level athlete to those outside of sport (Galli & Reel). For adolescent and college-aged athletes, an internal conflict can result from the dual pressure to conform to the often contrasting body standards of society and sport (Galli & Reel; Krane, Choi, Baird, Aimar, & Kauer, 2004). For female athletes, the conflict occurs due to participation in sports requiring higher muscle mass, which is in contrast to societal ideals demanding a skinny, yet toned, physique. For male athletes, weight training for muscle size and sym-metry is contrary to the goal of functional strength for sport performance. Both sport-specific and general societal weight- and body-related pressure are key components of Petrie and Greenleaf's (2007; 2012) etiological model of eating disorders in athletes, and the results of several large-scale cross-sectional inves-tigations support athletes' perceptions of weight and body pressure as related to body image and disordered eating in male and female athletes (Galli, Petrie, Reel, Baghurst, & Chatterton, 2014; Galli, Petrie, Reel, Greenleaf, & Carter, 2015; Reel, Petrie, SooHoo, & Anderson, 2013).

Weight-class sports are notorious for supporting a sub-culture in which "cutting" large amounts of weight in a short period of time is not only accepted but encouraged. The peer pressure to cut weight was on worldwide display in the fifth season of the television show *The Ultimate Fighter*, in which hopeful UFC fighter Gabe Ruediger was kicked off the show after failing to make weight for an upcoming fight. Prior to being removed, Ruediger, who was 20 pounds over the weight limit for his fight, is depicted receiving a colonic, and requesting that his coach and teammates literally drag him back into a sauna to resume exercising and sweat off excess weight. Ruediger's former teammates and coaches are later seen questioning his dedication to the sport. The experience of Ruediger and many others can be explained by the sense of belonging, professionalism, and prestige displayed when athletes in weight-class sports make the sacrifice to cut weight (Pettersson, Ekström, & Berg, 2013). As one combat-sport athlete put it, "If you didn't cut at least 7 kilos you were considered …. bad … you were not considered as a serious athlete" (Pettersson et al., p. 102). Thus, the culture of weight cutting in combat and other weight-class sports, in which rapid weight loss behaviors are a symbol of dedication and professionalism, serve as a source of psychological pressure for athletes in these sports to engage in potentially unsafe weight-cutting practices such as caloric restriction and excessive exercise.

Aesthetic sport athletes such as gymnasts, divers, and figure skaters are yet another group of individuals who often experience intense pressure to alter their body. Weight/body pressure for athletes in aesthetic sports is twofold: (a) due to the importance of being explosive, agile, and flexible, the potential performance advantage conferred by maintaining a certain (often lighter) body weight, and (b) a sub-culture that has long valued and promoted a light and lean body frame. Athletes in aesthetic sports consistently report lower body satisfaction and more disordered eating compared to athletes in other sports (e.g., Byrne & McLean, 2002; Krentz & Warschburger, 2013).

Coaches in aesthetic sports seem to have a particularly powerful influence, as most athletes report feeling weight- and/or body-related pressure from their coaches (Kong & Harris, 2015). Qualitative interviews have shed light on the context for and experience of weight- and body-related pressures for these athletes. A key finding across studies and interviews with current and former parents, athletes, and judges, is the notion of control. One parent of a gymnast reported her concerns about the degree of control her daughter's coach had over weight monitoring:

> After learning that my daughter was underweight for her age, I told the coach the constant weighing had to stop. But the coaches want all control and the parents are to have none. I would not encourage my grandchildren or anyone else to go into this sport unless I saw a great change in the coaching style.
>
> *(Kerr, Berman, & De Souza, 2006, p. 33)*

Figure skaters in a study by Voelker and Reel (2015) noted similarly controlling practices by their coaches. A few quotes from this study stand out as particularly powerful. "I remember they would bring out the scale and once a week they would have weigh-ins. Everybody could see it … and it was run by the coaches." "If you're at the rink and eating junk food, the coaches will go insane and be like 'Oh my God what are you doing?!'" "I've seen coaches who make you keep a journal of everything you eat, have a certain number of calories that you can eat per day … what you're allowed to eat and what you're not" (p. 303). Galli and

Reel (2009) found that male athletes are not immune to weight/body pressure from coaches. One collegiate American football player offered an in-depth description of how his coach pressured him to gain weight:

> I weigh in once at the beginning of the week and end of the week ... there's a punishment if you don't make your weight, because he's been telling you for so long, "You have to make your weight".... They'll make you come in at 6:30 a.m. and drink water and protein shakes until you're at your weight.
>
> *(p. 101)*

The lengths coaches go to in order to control athletes' weight and eating behaviors not only undermine athletes' autonomy but can also normalize pathological behaviors such as self-starvation, excessive exercise, and substance abuse.

Summary

In addition to the typical psychological pressure to perform that is present for all high-level athletes, those athletes in sports emphasizing endurance or aesthetics, or with a designated weight requirement, face additional psychological pressure to conform to certain body-weight and appearance standards. These pressures can originate from a variety of sources, but are often perpetuated by the unique, and often misguided, sub-culture of leanness-focused sports. Coaches are a particularly powerful source of pressure, and may encourage athletes to engage in unhealthy and unsafe body-change behaviors.

Future research directions

As researchers become more consumed with the question of how athletes perform in acute pressure-packed situations, the psychosocial health consequences of chronic, day-to-day pressure encountered by high-level athletes seems less of a priority. Perhaps it's because addressing such pressure necessarily requires a critical analysis of business-as-usual practices of elite sport organizations that prioritize winning over well-being. As was done by Coker-Cranney, Watson, Bernstein, Voelker, & Coakley (2018) when studying deviant overconformity in wrestlers, there is a need for researchers to examine the antecedents and consequences of psychological pressure for high-level athletes from the perspective of relevant sociological theories of high-level sport. In doing so, researchers will need to commit to methods that go beyond self-report paper-and-pencil questionnaires and include in-depth interviews, focus groups, and ethnographic inquiries that allow for a richer and more nuanced understanding of high-level athletes' experience of pressure. Such investigations would necessarily offer a more holistic view of the nature of psychological pressure in high-level sport by including the perceptions of parents, coaches, and sport administrators.

Traditional quantitative investigations will remain important, but it is only through prospective and longitudinal designs that researchers will distinguish between athletes who adapt well to high-level sport environments and those who experience adverse psychosocial health outcomes. Longitudinal case studies with athletes as they advance through the developmental pipeline would offer valuable insight into the evolution of pressure for high-level athletes. Finally, professional athletes who compete in high-profile sports and under constant media pressure remain understudied, and efforts should be made to include these individuals in future investigations.

Conclusion

From elite youth to professional-level competition, high-level athletes operate under constant expectations of success from family, coaches, media, and others. When performance-based expectations are not balanced with consideration for the health, well-being, and personal development of athletes, and/or when athletes lack effective coping skills, the ensuing psychological pressure does not bode well for athletes' psychosocial health and well-being. Sociological theories of deviance and burnout in sport are instructive for the issue of psychological pressure in sport, and implicate the win-at-all-cost nature of high-level sport organizations for creating a culture in which athletes are expected to overextend themselves and do whatever it takes to win. Athletes in sports where body weight, shape, and size are of primary concern face additional pressure to conform to the accepted body standards of their sport. Although the nature and source of pressure change as high-level athletes develop and advance, athletes who experience extreme psychological pressure at any level may become less satisfied with sport, feel worse about themselves, have relationship difficulties, and feel compelled to engage in a variety of unhealthy practices such as disordered eating and substance abuse. Researchers who wish to learn more about general psychological pressure for high-level athletes should consider adopting a socio-psychological approach to this issue, in which pressure is viewed as a manifestation of the high-level sport culture rather than simply a failure of athletes to adequately cope with demands.

References

Amorose, A. J., & Anderson-Butcher, D. (2015). Exploring the independent and interactive effects of autonomy-supportive and controlling coaching behaviors on adolescent athletes' motivation for sport. *Sport, Exercise, and Performance Psychology, 4*(3), 206–218. doi:10.1037/spy0000038

Amorose, A. J., Anderson-Butcher, D., Newman, T. J., Fraina, M., & Iachini, A. (2016). High school athletes' self-determined motivation: The independent and interactive effects of coach, father, and mother autonomy support. *Psychology of Sport and Exercise, 26*, 1–8. doi:10.1016/j.psychsport.2016.05.005

Battaglia, A. V., Kerr, G., & Stirling, A. E. (2017). Youth athletes' interpretations of punitive coaching practices. *Journal of Applied Sport Psychology, 29*(3), 337–352. doi:10.1080/10413200.2016.1271370

Byrne, S., & McLean, N. (2002). Elite athletes: Effects of the pressure to be thin. *Journal of Science & Medicine in Sport, 5*(2), 80–94.

Coakley, J. (1992). Burnout among adolescent athletes: A personal failure or social problem? *Sociology of Sport Journal, 9*(3), 271–285.

Coker-Cranney, A., Watson, J. C., II, Bernstein, M., Voelker, D. K., & Coakley, J. (2018). How far is too far? Understanding identity and overconformity in collegiate wrestlers. *Qualitative Research in Sport, Exercise and Health*. doi:10.1080/2159676X.2017.1372798

Cooper, J. N., & Cooper, J. E. (2015). "I'm running so you can be happy and I can keep my scholarship": A comparative study of Black male college athletes' experiences with role conflict. *Journal of Intercollegiate Sport, 8*(2), 131–152. doi:10.1123/jis.2014-0120

Deci, E. L., & Ryan, R. M. (1985). *Intrinsic motivation and self-determination in human behavior*. New York, NY: Plenum.

Donovan, L. (2013). *Landon Donovan on the stress of being a professional athlete*. Retrieved from https://www.huffingtonpost.com/2013/05/16/landon-donovan-stress-mental-exhaustion_n_3286913.html

Dunn, R. C., Dorsch, T. E., King, M. Q. & Rothlisberger, K. J. (2016). The impact of family financial investment on perceived parent pressure and child enjoyment and commitment in organized youth sport. *Family Relations: An Interdisciplinary Journal of Applied Family Studies, 65*(2), 287–299. doi:10.1111/fare.12193

Galli, N., Petrie, T. A., Reel, J. J., Chatterton, J. M., & Baghurst, T. M. (2014). Assessing the validity of the weight pressures in sport scale for male athletes. *Psychology of Men & Masculinity, 15*(2), 170–180. doi:10.1037/a0031762

Galli, N., Petrie, T. A., Reel, J. J., Greenleaf, C., & Carter, J. E. (2015). Psychosocial predictors of drive for muscularity in male collegiate athletes. *Body Image, 14*, 62–66. doi:10.1016/j.bodyim.2015.03.009

Galli. N., & Reel, J. J. (2009). Adonis or Hephaestus? Exploring body image in male athletes. *Psychology of Men & Masculinity, 10*(2), 95–108.

Gould, D., Lauer, L., Rolo, C., Jannes, C., & Pennisi, N, (2006). Understanding the role parents play in tennis success: A national survey of junior tennis coaches. *British Journal of Sports Medicine, 40*(7), 632–638. doi:10.1136/bjsm.2005.024927

Harkness, R. (2017). *Dana White: Jon Jones couldn't handle the pressure of being champ*. Retrieved from https://www.mmamania.com/2017/10/9/16449046/dana-white-fame-and-fortune-defeated-jon-jones

Hickey, C., & Kelly, P. (2008). Preparing to not be a footballer: Higher education and professional sport. *Sport, Education and Society, 13*(4), 477–494. doi:10.1080/13573320802445132

Hill, D. M., Carvell, S., Matthews, N., Weston, N. J. V., & Thelwell, R. C. C. (2017). Exploring choking experiences in elite sport: The role of self-presentation. *Psychology of Sport and Exercise, 33*, 141–149. doi:10.1037/t20676-000

Hughes, R., & Coakley, J. (1991). Positive deviance among athletes: The implications of overconformity to the sport ethic. *Sociology of Sport Journal, 8*(4), 307–325.

Jõesaar, H., Hein, V., & Hagger, M. S. (2012). Youth athletes' perception of autonomy support from the coach, peer motivational climate and intrinsic motivation in sport setting: One-year effects. *Psychology of Sport and Exercise, 13*(3), 257–262. doi:10.1016/j.psychsport.2011.12.001

Kerr, G., Berman, E., & De Souza, M. J. (2006). Disordered eating in women's gymnastics: Perspectives of athletes, coaches, parents, and judges. *Journal of Applied Sport Psychology, 18*(1), 28–43. doi:10.1080/10413200500471301

Kimball, A., & Freysinger, V. J. (2003). 15. Leisure, stress, and coping: The sport participation of collegiate student-athletes. *Leisure Sciences, 25*(2–3), 115–141. doi:10.1080/01490400306569

Kong, P., & Harris, L. M. (2015). The sporting body: Body image and eating disorder symptomatology among female athletes from leanness focused and nonleanness focused sports. *Journal of Psychology, 149*(2), 141–160. doi:10.1080/00223980.2013.846291

Krane, V., Choi, P. Y. L., & Baird, S. M. (2004). Living the paradox: Female athletes negotiate femininity and muscularity. *Sex Roles, 50*(5/6), 315–329. doi:10.1023/B:SERS.0000018888.48437.4f

Krentz, E. M., & Warschburger, P. (2013). A longitudinal investigation of sports-related risk factors for disordered eating in aesthetic sports. *Scandinavian Journal of Medicine & Science in Sports, 23*(3), 303–310. doi:10.1111/j.1600-0838.2011.01380.x

Mayer, J., & Thiel, A. (2018). Presenteeism in the elite sports workplace: The willingness to compete hurt among German elite handball and track and field athletes. *International Review for the Sociology of Sport, 53*(1), 49–68. doi:10.1177/1012690216640525

McCarthy, P. J., & Jones, M. V. (2007). A qualitative study of sport enjoyment in the sampling years. *The Sport Psychologist, 21*(4), 400–416.

McKay, J., Niven, A. A., Lavallee, D., & White, A. (2008). Sources of strain among elite UK track athletes. *The Sport Psychologist, 22*, 143–163.

Messner, M. A. (1995). *Power at play: Sports and the problem of masculinity.* Boston, MA: Beacon Press.

Ohl, F., Fincoeur, B., Lentillon-Kaestner, V., Defrance, J., & Brissonneau, C. (2015). The socialization of young cyclists and the culture of doping. *International Review for the Sociology of Sport, 50*(7), 865–882. doi;10.1177/1012690213495534

Parsons, J. (2013). Student athlete perceptions of academic success and athlete stereotypes on campus. *Journal of Sport Behavior, 36*(4), 400–416.

Paule, A. L., & Gilson, T. A. (2010). Current collegiate experiences of big-time, non-revenue, NCAA athletes. *Journal of Intercollegiate Sport, 3*(2), 333–347. doi:10.1123/jis.3.2.333

Petrie, T. A., & Greenleaf, C. (2012). Eating disorders in sport. In S. M. Murphy (Ed.), *The Oxford handbook of sport and performance psychology* (pp. 635–659). New York, NY: Oxford University Press.

Petrie, T. A., & Greenleaf, C. A. (2007). Eating disorders in sport: From theory to research to intervention. In G. Tenenbaum & R. C. Eklund (Eds.), *Handbook of sport psychology* (3rd ed., pp. 352–378). Hoboken, NJ: John Wiley & Sons.

Pettersson, S., Ekström, M., & Berg, C. (2013). Practices of weight regulation among elite athletes in combat sports: A matter of mental advantage? *Journal of Athletic Training, 48*, 99–108. doi:10.4085/1062-6050-48.1.04.

Reel, J. J., & Gill, D. L. (2001). Slim enough to swim? Weight pressures for competitive swimmers and coaching implications. *The Sport Journal.* Retrieved from http://thesportjournal.org/article/slim-enough-to-swim-weight-pressures-for-competitive-swimmers-and-coaching-implications/

Reel, J. J., Petrie, T. A., Soohoo, S., Anderson, C. M. (2013). Weight pressures in sport: Examining the factor structure and incremental validity of the weight pressures in sport—Females. *Eating Behaviors, 14*(2), 137–144. doi:10.1016/j.eatbeh.2013.01.003

Rhatigan, J. J. (1984). Serving two masters: The plight of the college student-athlete. *New Directions for Student Services, 1984*(28), 5–11. doi:10.1002/ss.37119842803

Rothschild-Checroune, E., Gravelle, F., Dawson, D., & Karlis, G. (2013). Balancing academic and athletic time management: A qualitative exploration of first year student athletes' university football experiences. *Society and Leisure. 35.* 243–261. doi:10.1080/07053436.2012.10707843

Sánchez-Miguel, P. A., Leo, F. M., Sánchez-Oliva, D., Amado, D., & García-Calvo, T. (2013). The importance of parents' behavior in their children's enjoyment and motivation in sports. *Journal of Human Kinetics, 36,* 169–177. doi:10.2478/hukin-2013-0017

Stebbings, J., Taylor, I. M., Spray, C. M., & Ntoumanis, N. (2012). Antecedents of perceived coach interpersonal behaviors: The coaching environment and coach psychological well- and ill-being. *Journal of Sport & Exercise Psychology, 34*(4), 481–502.

Swann, C., Crust, L., Jackman, P., Vella, S. A., Allen, M. S., & Keegan, R. (2017). Performing under pressure: Exploring the psychological state underlying clutch performance in sport. *Journal of Sports Sciences, 35*(23), 2272–2280. doi:10.1080/02640414.2016.1265661

Vaz, E. V. (1974). What price victory? An analysis of minor hockey league players' attitudes toward winning. *International Review of Sport Sociology, 9*(2), 33–35.

Voelker, D. K., & Galli, N. (in press). *APA handbook of sport and exercise psychology.* Washington: American Psychological Association.

Voelker, D. K., & Reel, J. J. (2015). An inductive thematic analysis of female competitive figure skaters' experiences of weight pressure in sport. *Journal of Clinical Sport Psychology, 9*(4), 297–316.

Waldron, J. J., & Krane, V. (2005). Whatever it takes: Health compromising behaviors in female athletes. *Quest, 57*(3), 315–329. doi:10.1080/00336297.2005.10491860

Wiese-Bjornstal, D. (2000). Playing with injury. *Athletic Therapy Today, 5*(2), 60–61.

6
ABUSE

James is a 13-year-old boy who plays American football in a high-profile youth league. Residents of the particular town where James lives are fanatical about football, and their enthusiasm is just as evident for the youth games played on Saturdays as it is for the professional games played on Sundays. In many ways, youth football is viewed as the minor league for local high-school and college teams, and parents are emotionally invested in the success of their children, as it could lead to a college scholarship, or perhaps even a lucrative professional contract. James' coach symbolizes the seriousness with which the game is taken. He is known to loudly berate players who fail to properly execute their assignment, and on occasion will kick and throw clipboards and other equipment during his tirades. James is the star running back, but unfortunately he had two costly fumbles in the last game. After enduring a particularly humiliating tongue lashing in front of his teammates after the game, James is eager to have a good week of practice leading to the next game. Upon arriving at practice on Monday, James is both hurt and surprised when his coach fails to offer any verbal feedback at all, and appears to intentionally avoid eye contact with him. After seeing the effect that the coach's behavior has on James, his parents have some concern about the coach's tactics. But after talking to other parents and observing the behavior of other coaches, they conclude that his behavior isn't overly unusual. In fact, the coach has won multiple league championships, and several of his former players have gone on to earn scholarships to play football collegiately. Because of the coach's track record, both James and his parents decide that James is best served by having a "thick skin," and earning his way back into the coach's favor by playing better next week.

One of the many benefits of sport participation is the opportunity to form satisfying relationships with peers, coaches, and others in the sport environment. When relationships are based on a foundation of trust and mutual respect, athletes are in a position not only to achieve their performance goals, but to reap psychosocial health benefits in the form of enhanced subjective, psychological, and social well-being. Unfortunately, high-level sport also presents the opportunity for dysfunctional and abusive relationships that can cause long-term psychosocial damage. At times, abuse is a case of coaches or administrators taking the "win-at-all-costs" mentality discussed in Chapter 5 to the extreme. As with James and his coach, on-field success can serve to justify abusive actions and mask the potential psychosocial harm caused by abusive behavior. Athlete abuse also occurs when individuals in positions of power decide to leverage this power to fulfill personal desires. Whatever the reasons, abuse represents perhaps the most insidious threat to athletes' psychosocial health.

Three recent examples highlight the dark side of relationships in high-level sport. First, former professional soccer player Andy Woodward came forward with accounts of sexual abuse by his youth coach. Following Woodward's revelation, several more British soccer players came forward with similar stories of abuse. In the 1970s, one player was allegedly paid £50,000 by Chelsea Football Club to remain silent about incidents of abuse. Second, the case of Dr. Larry Nassar, the longtime USA Gymnastics and Michigan State University physician who sexually abused hundreds of athletes between 1992 and 2015 (Joseph, 2018). Although these cases represent perhaps the worst possible scenario of abuse in high-level sport settings, emotional and sexual abuse are unfortunately not uncommon. In rare cases, abuse can lead to a fatality. A University of Maryland football player passed away following a team workout in June 2018. Following an investigation, a culture of verbal and physical abuse was revealed, including weights being thrown at players, mocking of players' masculinity when unable to complete a workout, and forced overeating to the point of vomiting as punishment.

In this chapter I begin by providing an overview of the general and sport-specific literature on the two most common types of abuse in high-level sport—sexual and verbal abuse. I draw from the extensive body of knowledge on parental abuse to define key terms and explain the underlying reasons for the occurrence of abusive behavior. As part of this discussion I highlight the potential psychosocial consequences for athletes who are victims of abuse. Finally, I suggest future research directions to enhance understanding of the causes, experience, and outcomes of abuse in high-level sport.

Much of what is known about abuse and abusive relationships comes from research on and clinician accounts of spousal and child abuse, in which individuals who hold power in the relationship engage in abusive behaviors to retain their control over another person. Although the exact reasons for abuse depend on the person and the situation, abusers were often abused themselves, and have come to believe that such behavior works to their benefit (Patricelli, 2018). Some abusers may also suffer from personality disorders such as borderline personality disorder (de Aquino Ferreira, Queiroz Pereira, Neri Benevides, & Aguiar Melo, 2018) or antisocial personality disorder (Billick & Jackson, 2007). Abuse can take many forms, including physical, financial, and spiritual, but two of the most common forms of abuse in high-level sport are emotional (aka psychological), and sexual (Mountjoy et al., 2016).

Emotional abuse in sport

Emotional abuse occurs when one party engages in a pattern of harmful, but physical contact-free, interactions with another party which cause extreme emotional discomfort (Glaser, 2002). Like most forms of abuse, emotional abuse tends to occur when one individual seeks to gain or retain control over another, and often takes the form of threats, humiliation, name-calling, and/or yelling (Tracy, 2016). Perhaps due to an implicit acceptance of behaviors associated with emotional abuse, and/or the perception that the perpetrators of such behaviors don't intend to harm others, emotional abuse has garnered less attention from researchers than other forms of abuse (Brassard & Donovan, 2006). Common settings for emotional abuse include romantic relationships (Dutton, Goodman, & Bennett, 1999), parent/caregiver-child relationships (Straus & Field, 2003), and the workplace (Keashley & Jagatic, 2010). Regardless of the setting, individuals subjected to chronic emotional abuse may experience adverse cognitive, emotional, and social outcomes (e.g., Reuben, et al., 2016). Within sport, the considerable power wielded by coaches to influence athletes' position on the team, playing opportunities, and connections with higher-level teams, makes the coach-athlete relationship a prime site for emotional abuse (Gervis & Dunn, 2004).

Coaches have long been known to employ emotional abuse in misguided attempts to motivate and cultivate mental toughness in athletes (Owusu-Sekyere & Gervis, 2016). Indeed, 12 out of 12 elite youth athletes interviewed by Owusu-Sekyre and Gervis (2016) noted that their coach frequently shouted at them, and 9 out of 12 reported that they were frequently belittled or humiliated by their coach. Emotional abuse may be even more common in individual sports such as gymnastics, swimming, and figure skating, in which competitors begin training at a young age and spend many hours each day in close contact with their coach. In response to the growing problem of overtraining and abuse in elite youth sport, Donnelly (1997) famously called for the application of child labor laws to this context. At Pennsylvania State University, a husband-wife pair of gymnastics coaches used threats and name calling to encourage athletes to lose weight (Dryball, 2016). After Thanksgiving break, one coach reportedly greeted the returning gymnasts with the following comment: "Wow, you guys look like you ate your way through break" (para. 10). Another gymnast was told that she was so fat that she "looked like a whale" (para. 11). Team sports are not immune to emotional abuse. Bob Knight, regarded as one of the greatest college basketball coaches of all time, was known to verbally and physically assault his players when he believed they lacked discipline on the court. Of his many famous quotes, one typifies his approach to coaching: "People want national championship banners. People want to talk about Indiana being competitive. How do we get there? We don't get there with milk and cookies" (Pace, 2012). The previous examples illustrate the line between challenge and abuse crossed when coaches blindly seek to "toughen athletes up" for the rigors of competition (Owusu-Sekyere & Gervis, 2016).

The uniqueness of high-level sport necessitates a context-driven definition of emotional abuse. Following interviews with 14 retired elite female swimmers, in which athletes described emotional abuse from coaches in the form of hitting or throwing objects (e.g., blocks), verbal aggression (e.g., "worthless," "disgusting"), and denial of attention and support (e.g., intentional lack of verbal interaction and eye contact), Stirling and Kerr (2008) proposed a sport-specific definition of emotional abuse. In addition to the aforementioned characteristics of (a) a pattern of behavior, (b) free from physical contact, (c) causing extreme emotional discomfort, the authors emphasized that emotional abuse occurs in the context of a critical relationship (e.g., coach-athlete), and highlight the various ways that emotional abuse can occur in the high-level sport-environment (e.g., physical, verbal, denial of service). Interestingly, denial of attention was viewed as the most disturbing method of emotional abuse. Because young athletes rely on their coaches for feedback and support for their success, a unique feature of emotional abuse in the sport context is the intentional withholding of information that could potentially enhance athletes' chances of learning and development. Gervis (2009) added further depth to the understanding of emotional abuse in sport in her process model. Central to the model is a sport culture characterized by an imbalance of power, extreme pressure to perform, and long hours of contact between athletes and coaches. Within such a culture, coaches may feel compelled to adopt abusive behaviors such as those described by athletes in the Stirling and Kerr (2008), which may have negative consequences for athletes' emotional health and on-field performance.

More recently, Stirling and Kerr (2013) proposed a holistic ecological model of athlete vulnerability to coach emotional abuse. Based both on the results of their own interviews, as well as non-sport models of child maltreatment, they constructed a circular four-level model. The outer circle encompasses the *macrosystem* supporting emotional abuse in sport, which in Western societies is characterized by a performance combined with media representations condoning coach abuse, and an overall cultural acceptance of violence and aggression. The next circle in the model describes the emotional abuse *exosystem*, which narrows the focus to elements of the sport community supporting emotional abuse, including shifting of control from parents to coaches, coach reputation, exposure to the emotional abuse of teammates, and inadequate institutional procedures for handling reports of abuse. The *microsystem* is the second most inner circle, and represents the daily interactions and overall relationship between athletes and coaches. Factors such as time spent together, athlete trust and respect for the coach, athlete performance, and timely praise from the coach can all set the stage for abusive behavior. Finally, in the innermost circle resides coaches' *ontological development*, which refers to characteristics and pre-dispositions that may support abusive practices, such as unrealistic expectations, poor emotional management, and a coaching philosophy in which abusive practices are considered a critical component of athlete development.

A hypothetical example of a teenage tennis player illustrates how Stirling and Kerr's (2013) ecological model may operate in practice. First, years of exposure to movies and television shows depicting fiery coaches inspiring athletes to succeed on and off the field help to both normalize and justify abusive coach behavior (the macrosystem of emotional abuse). Second, upon achieving success locally, the athlete and her family may decide it best for her to move away from home to pursue specialized training at an elite tennis academy. She may be thrust into a training environment in which coaches exert complete control over players, with few consequences for abusive behavior. Far from home, and a newcomer to the system, it becomes easy for the player to accept and internalize the norms of her new training environment as being necessary for goal achievement (i.e., the exosystem of emotional abuse). Within the context of this macro and exosystem, the athlete develops a relationship with her new coach that is fortified by the athlete's admiration for the accomplishments of the coach, as well as the considerable time spent together in training (i.e., the microsystem of emotional abuse). The macro-, exo-, and microsystem further reinforce the coach's "tough love" approach to coaching learned from his coaches (i.e., the ontological development of the abuser), and offer him the latitude to shout, belittle, intimidate, and/or ignore the player whenever he sees fit.

As with other threats to athlete psychosocial health, and as Stirling and Kerr's (2013) model suggests, abusive behavior is a byproduct of sport institutions that value winning over personal development, and administrators who are willing to ignore coach transgressions in the name of performance. Emotional abuse is often justified, so long as it supports the goals of winning, and is free of violent physical contact with athletes (Jacobs, Smits, & Knoppers, 2017). In one study, directors of elite women's gymnastics clubs normalized abusive coaching practices by suggesting that such behaviors are a natural trade-off for having an elite club, and that placing more emphasis on personal development would prevent them from hiring the best coaches. As one director said,

> Elite sport is about winning. That characterizes elite sport. The moment you say that is not so, then there is nothing left to talk about. If you say to your coach that winning is unimportant and that pleasure or development are more important, than that elite coach will leave your club.
>
> (Jacobs et al., 2017, p. 131)

Directors in this study also laid blame on parents. "[Parents] do not come because you promise a child friendly or child focused programs. No, people who want elite sport do not come for that; they come because they want to win" (Jacobs et al., 2017, p. 134). It seems that coaches and directors struggle to envision a gray area in which sport organizations work to enhance both athlete development and performance in an integrated way, rather than treat them as paradoxical outcomes.

Summary

The imbalance of power existing between athletes and coaches, coupled with regular and lengthy periods of contact, make high-level sport a prime context for emotional abuse. Emotional abuse from coaches can take the form of physical actions (e.g., breaking a clipboard), verbal aggression (e.g., name-calling), and/or the denial of support (e.g., ignoring an athlete who performed below expectations). As coaches work to develop mentally tough athletes, the line between challenge and abuse may be crossed. The culture of sport, with its emphasis on performance over personal development, allows abusive behavior to be normalized rather than addressed as a problem.

Sexual abuse in sport

Sexual abuse, defined as unwanted sexual behavior from one person to another, is a serious public health issue worldwide. For example, the lifetime prevalence of sexual abuse among U.S. women is 18%, with most (75%) incidents of abuse perpetrated by individuals known to the victim (Truman, 2011). As with emotional abuse, sexual abuse often occurs in the context of a relationship in which one person is in a position of power over another. Thus, women, children, the elderly, and people with cognitive disabilities are often victims of sexual abuse.

Several theories have been proposed to explain sexual abuse in general, including those focused on biology (Hucker & Bain, 1990), cognition (Ward & Keenan, 1999), and social learning (Laws & Marshall, 1990). However, owing to the complexity of sexual abuse, multi-factor theories such as Marshall and Barbaree's (1990) Integrated Theory, and Stinson, Sales and Becker's (2008) Multimodal Self-Regulation Theory have garnered favor. Although no single theory has emerged as superior, in her review of the etiology of sexual abuse, Faupel and Pryzbylski (2017) highlighted several factors consistently linked to it, including adverse childhood conditions, perceived costs/benefits of abusive behaviors, distorted patterns of thinking, repeated exposure to violent pornography, poor self-regulation and impulse control, and low empathy.

Because of the hierarchical nature of relationships in high-level sport (e.g., coach-athlete, support staff-athlete, older athlete-younger athlete), these environments are ripe for the occurrence of sexual abuse. In addition to the imbalance of power between adults in positions of authority and young athletes, the unique norms of sport, in which adult coaches are often given free rein to physically touch, maneuver, or adjust athletes, may blur the lines between proper instruction and abuse (Tschan, 2013). As seen in the cases of the young English soccer players and the U.S. gymnasts abused by Larry Nassar described at the beginning of this chapter, much of the sexual abuse in high-level sport occurs within elite youth sport.

In a large retrospective study with over 6,000 collegiate athletes in the United Kingdom, 29% reported being sexually abused as youth athletes—a much higher prevalence of abuse than among children in the general population (Alexander, Stafford, & Lewis, 2011). Further findings by Alexander et al. (2011) showed that whereas teammates were more often the perpetrators of sexual abuse at lower levels of sport, coaches more commonly committed sexual abuse at higher levels. Most perpetrators of sexual abuse in sport are male coaches (Vertommen, Schipper-Van Veldhoven, Hartill, & Van Den Eede, 2015), and victims are more often girls and from ethnic minority groups (Bjørnseth & Szabo, 2018). However, despite experiencing sexual abuse at lower rates than female athletes, male athletes are certainly not immune to the problem. In one study of Australian athletes, 21% of male athletes reported having been sexually abused, with 29% of these athletes reporting that the abuse occurred in the sport environment (Leahy, Pretty, & Tenenbaum, 2002).

A key feature of sexual abuse in youth sport is the process of *grooming*, in which coaches, staff, or more senior athletes intentionally forge close emotional bonds with a target with the purpose of lowering their inhibition to engage in sexual contact (Brackenridge & Fasting, 2005). The perpetrators of sexual abuse in sport (often coaches) systematically set the stage for sexual contact with young athletes by building trust and friendship, establishing loyalty, and upon initiation of sexual abuse, ensuring the secrecy of these acts (Cense & Brackenridge, 2001). To expose the multiple meanings of the grooming process in sport through the voice of a victim, Owton and Sparkes (2017) undertook a collaborative autoethnography alongside a female athlete with the pseudonym Bella. Through analysis of poems and stories created and shared by Bella, Owton and Sparkes represented her perceptions of the grooming process that led to being sexually abused by her coach. Her stories illustrate the grooming tactics of targeting and trust building described by Brackenridge. In brief, Bella discussed how her coach targeted her based on her slight build, newness to the team, and troubled home life. The coach worked to build trust and loyalty by buying Bella and her teammate alcoholic beverages and waiting with her for her mother after practice. Bella described providing her coach with foot massages, and her coach using this as an opportunity to "reciprocate" by giving her a massage for her back. To isolate and gain access to Bella, the coach invited her over for sleepovers at his home. Overall, Bella's story as represented by Owton and Sparkes offers an in-depth account of the grooming process that all too often occurs in elite youth sport, and shows how adults in the sport environment can rather easily use their position of authority to disadvantage and abuse vulnerable sport participants.

Although regardless of how it is handled, sexual abuse is a risk factor for negative psychosocial health, the consequences are even more debilitative when athletes feel uncomfortable disclosing that they have been abused (Lange, de Beurs, Dolan, Lachnit, Sjollema, & Hanewald, 1999). Athletes may fail to report instances of sexual abuse for several reasons, including fear of retribution from others, fear of being ostracized, the belief that others will not believe or defend them, or the belief that sexual behaviors on the part of coaches or others are a normal and appropriate part of the sport environment (Stirling & Kerr, 2009). In an analysis of the processes used by high-level Canadian sport organizations in responding to cases of sexual abuse, Parent (2011) found several issues that could impede disclosure and proper reporting. For example, athletes indicated reluctance to report sexual abuse to administrators due to the perception that the administrator and perpetrator (often a coach) were friends, and in some instances, administrators admitted to not knowing the signs of sexual abuse, nor the proper procedures for handling such reports. From a positive perspective, administrators noted how dealing with a case of sexual abuse prompted them to subsequently become more preventive and proactive regarding the issue.

Summary

Recent media reports, as well as a growing body of research, highlight sexual abuse as a serious threat to the psychosocial health and well-being of athletes. Sexual abuse is at least as common, and perhaps more so, among children who play sport versus children in general. As with emotional abuse, elements of the high-level sport environment, including power imbalance and contact time, present the opportunity for sexual abuse to occur. Further, norms of sport supporting physical contact between coaches and athletes may blur the line between appropriate and inappropriate coach-athlete interactions. Coaches and other adults in positions of power systematically groom athletes for abuse, and once abuse occurs, many organizations are ill-equipped to handle allegations of sexual abuse.

Psychosocial health consequences of abuse in sport

Depending on the duration and severity, abuse in any form can be a traumatic life experience for the victim. Indeed, both emotional and sexual abuse are listed as two types of trauma by the National Traumatic Stress Network. For both athletes and non-athletes, abuse has the potential to adversely affect all four aspects of psychosocial health. In terms of emotional health, substantial evidence in the general psychology literature links abuse to a variety of concerns, including anxiety (Banducci, Lejuez, Dougherty, & MacPherson, 2017), depression (Gibb, Chelminski, & Zimmerman, 2007), and posttraumatic stress (Collings, 2012). Further, victims of emotional and sexual abuse are at risk of engaging in unhealthy behaviors such as substance abuse and disordered eating (Afifi, Henriksen, Asmundson & Sareen, 2012; Brener, McMahon, Warren, & Douglas, 1999). Although less is known about how abuse affects other domains of psychosocial health, findings indicate that abuse may be directly or indirectly related to cognitive deficits (Vasilevski & Tucker, 2015), poorer social functioning (McCaw, Golding, Farley, & Minkoff, 2007), and less spirituality (Sansone, Kelley, & Forbis, 2013).

In addition to the general psychosocial impairments experienced by all victims of abuse, athletes who suffer abuse in the sport context also experience impairments specific to that environment. Athletes interviewed for studies of emotional abuse described feeling upset, scared, angry, anxious, as well as experiencing damage to their body image and self-esteem (Stirling & Kerr, 2008; 2013). Motivation and enjoyment for sport may also decrease, as athletes eventually tire of coaches' abusive language and behavior (Stirling & Kerr, 2013). From the perspective of cognitive health, some athletes discussed difficulty focusing and acquiring new skills under conditions of emotional abuse. One interesting finding was that some athletes perceived *benefits* for their motivation and sense of accomplishment due to emotional abuse from their coach. The latter finding may speak to the extent to which athletes internalize and come to accept abusive behaviors as a normal and acceptable part of the sport culture. Perhaps due to the difficulty in securing participants to report on such sensitive matters, compared to emotional abuse, the psychosocial consequences of sexual abuse in the high-level sport context are less understood. The limited research that is available suggests that athlete survivors of sexual abuse are likely to feel embarrassed, guilt at complying with the perpetrator, and because of the close bond formed with the perpetrator during the grooming process, a sense of self-blame at allowing the abuse to happen (Hartill, 2014).

Future research directions

Much work remains to eradicate emotional and sexual abuse from high-level sport. Quality research will assist policy makers in creating safe environments for athletes to achieve their potential as people and as athletes. Boys and young men remain underrepresented in studies of abuse in sport (Parent & Bannon, 2012). The culture of hyper-masculinity in high-level sport supports a "tough love" approach to feedback from coaches, and physical contact as a means of positive feedback for male athletes (e.g., slap on the behind, bear hug). Disclosure of abuse may be more difficult for boys and men, as doing so could be viewed as a sign of mental weakness. Further, because masculine norms dictate that "real men" are heterosexual, boys may be reluctant to report sexual abuse from their male coach out of fear of being labeled as gay. Thus, further research with male athletes is needed to better understand their perceptions of potentially abusive coach and teammate behavior.

Researchers have done well to reveal the prevalence and experience of abuse in sport. Although some research details the short-term emotional impact of abuse, less is known about the long-term psychosocial outcomes of abuse for athletes and former athletes, and how personality and other elements of the sport environment moderate such outcomes. For example, does competing as part of a sport organization with strong policies related to allegations of abuse ameliorate some of the negative effects of abuse? In doing so, researchers might consider testing general theoretical models of abuse and maltreatment discussed previously, and eventually modifying these for sport. Of course, it seems that most sport organizations are ill-equipped to handle abuse among their staff, and there is a need for more and better training programs related to best practices for handling abuse. Such programs should be properly evaluated using randomized controlled research designs that allow for causal inference regarding their effectiveness in preventing abuse and/or swiftly handling allegations of abuse. The USOC's Safe Sport program is an example of one such program in need of proper evaluation.

Conclusion

Recent high-profile cases highlight the pervasiveness of abusive behavior in high-level sport. When left unchecked, characteristics of the high-level sport environment such as an emphasis on performance over personal development, an imbalance of power between athletes and adult decision-makers, and long hours of contact, can set the stage for emotional and sexual abuse. Coaches, whether knowingly or inadvertently, often employ emotionally abusive tactics to control, motivate, and mentally toughen their athletes. Unfortunately, because the line between challenge and abuse is often unrecognizable to coaches, athletes, and parents, coaches can continue using such methods without repercussions. This may be especially true in circumstances where the coach has had success on the field of play, further justifying his methods. As opposed to emotional abuse, which often happens publicly, sexual abuse occurs behind the scenes with athletes who are compelled to remain silent. The perpetrators, often male coaches, groom vulnerable athletes for sexual contact by gaining their trust and then strategically isolating them from the rest of the team for personal attention. Many athletes fail to disclose incidents of sexual abuse out of embarrassment, guilt, shame, and a sense of loyalty to the perpetrator. Further research is needed to better understand the experiences of male athletes who have experienced abuse, to learn about the long-term psychosocial consequences of abuse for athletes, and to test the efficacy of abuse-prevention programs for sport.

References

Afifi, T. O., Henriksen, C. A., Asmundson, G. J., & Sareen, J. (2012). Childhood maltreatment and substance use disorders among men and women in a nationally representative sample. *The Canadian Journal of Psychiatry, 57*(11), 677–686. doi:10.1177/070674371205701105

Alexander, K., Stafford, A., & Lewis, R. (2011). The experiences of children participating in organised sport in the UK. London, United Kingdom: National Society for the Prevention of Cruelty to Children.

Banducci, A. N., Lejuez, C. W., Dougherty, L. R., & MacPherson, L. (2017). A prospective examination of the relations between emotional abuse and anxiety: Moderation by distress tolerance. *Prevention Science, 18*(1), 20–30. doi:10.1007/s11121-016-0691-y

Billick, S. B., & Jackson, M. B. (2007). Evaluating parents in child custody and abuse cases and the utility of psychological measures in screening for parental psychopathy or antisocial personality. In A. R. Felthous & S. Henning (Eds.), *International handbook on psychopathic disorders and the law* (Vol. 2, pp. 95–112). New York, NY: John Wiley & Sons.

Bjørnseth, I., & Szab, A. (2018). Sexual violence against children in sports and exercise: A systematic literature review. *Journal of Child Sexual Abuse, 27*(4), 365–385, doi:10.1 080/10538712.2018.1477222

Brackenridge, C., & Fasting, K. (2005). The grooming process in sport: Narratives of sexual harassment and abuse. *Auto/Biography, 13*(1), 33–52. doi:10.1191/0967550705 ab016oa

Brassard, M. R., & Donovan, K. L. (2006). Defining psychological maltreatment. In M. M. Freerick, J. F. Knutson, P. K. Trickett, & S. M. Flanzer (Eds.), *Child abuse and neglect: Definitions, classifications, and a framework for research* (pp. 151–197). Baltimore, MD: Paul H. Brookes.

Brener, N. D., McMahon, P. M., Warren, C. W., & Douglas, K. A. (1999). Forced sexual intercourse and associated health-risk behaviors among female college students in the United States. *Journal of Consulting and Clinical Psychology, 67,* 252–259. doi:10.1037/0022-006X.67.2.252

Cense, M., & Brackenridge, C. (2001). Temporal and developmental risk factors for sexual harassment and abuse in sport. *European Physical Education Review, 7*(1), 61–79. doi:10.1177/1356336X010071006

Collings, S. J. (2012). Child sexual abuse experiences mediate the relationship between poverty and posttraumatic stress disorder. *Social Behavior and Personality, 40*(6), 983–984.

de Aquino Ferreira, L. F., Queiroz Pereira, F. H., Neri Benevides, A. M. L., & Aguiar Melo, M. C. (2018). Borderline personality disorder and sexual abuse: A systematic review. *Psychiatry Research, 262,* 70–77. doi:10.1016/j.psychres.2018.01.043

Donnelly, P. (1997). Child labour, sport labour: Applying child labour laws to sport. *International Review for the Sociology of Sport, 32*(4), 389–406. doi:10.1177/101269097032004004

Dryball, R. (2016, May 31). *Penn State gymnasts allege emotional abuse, body-shaming against coaches: "They took everything away from me."* Retrieved form https://people.com/sports/ penn-state-womens-gymnastics-coaches-accused-of-emotional-abuse-body-shaming/

Dutton, M. A., Goodman, L. A., & Bennett, L. (1999). Court-involved battered women's responses to violence: The role of psychological, physical, and sexual abuse. *Violence and Victims, 14,* 89–104.

Faupel, S., & Przybylski, R. (2017). *Chapter 2: Etiology of adult sexual offending.* Office of Justice Programs, Sex Offender Management Assessment and Planning Initiative. Retrieved from https://smart.gov/SOMAPI/sec1/ch2_etiology.html

Gervis, M. (2009). *An investigation into the emotional responses of child athletes to their coach's behaviour from a child maltreatment perspective* (Unpublished master's thesis). Brunel University, London, United Kingdom.

Gervis, M., & Dunn, N. (2004). The emotional abuse of elite child athletes by their coaches. *Child Abuse Review, 13,* 215–223. doi:10.1002/car.843

Gibb, B. E., Chelminski, I., & Zimmerman, M. (2007). Childhood emotional, physical, and sexual abuse, and diagnoses of depressive and anxiety disorders in adult psychiatric outpatients. *Depression and Anxiety, 24,* 256–263. doi:10.1002/da.20238

Glaser, D. (2002). Emotional abuse and neglect (psychological maltreatment): A conceptual framework. *Child Abuse & Neglect, 26*, 697–714. doi:10.1016/S0145-2134(02)00342-3

Hucker, S., & Bain, J. (1990). Androgenic hormones and sexual assault. In W. L. Marshall & D. R. Laws (Eds.), *Handbook of sexual assault: Issues, theories and treatment of the offender* (pp. 93–102). New York, NY: Plenum Press.

Jacobs, F., Smits, F., & Knoppers, A. (2017). "You don't realize what you see!" The institutional context of emotional abuse in elite youth sport. *Sport in Society, 20*(1), 126–143. doi:10.1080/17430437.2015.1124567

Joseph, E. (2018, July 25). *Former USA Gymnastics doctor wants to be resentenced, disqualify judge who gave him 40–175 years in prison.* Retrieved from https://www.cnn.com/2018/07/25/us/michigan-larry-nassar/index.html

Keashly, L., & Jagatic, K (2010). North American perspectives on workplace hostility and bullying. In S. Einarsen, H. Hoel, & D. Zapf (Eds.), *Bullying and harassment in the workplace: Developments in theory, research and practice* (2nd ed., pp. 41–71). London, United Kingdom: Taylor Francis.

Lange, A., De Beurs, E., Dolan, C., Lachnit, T., Sjollema, S., & Hanewald, G. (1999). Objective and subjective characteristics of the abuse and psychopathology in later life. *The Journal of Nervous and Mental Disease, 187*(3), 150–158.

Laws, D. R., & Marshall, W. L. (1990). A conditioning theory of the etiology and maintenance of deviant sexual preference and behavior. In W. L. Marshall, D. R. Laws, & H. E. Barbaree (Eds.), *Handbook of sexual assault: Issues, theories, and treatment of the offender* (pp. 209–230). New York, NY: Plenum Press.

Leahy, T., Pretty, G., & Tenenbaum, G. (2002). Prevalence of sexual abuse in organised competitive sport in Australia. *Journal of Sexual Aggression, 8*(2), 16–36, doi:10.1080/13552600208413337

Marshall, W. L., & Barbaree, H. E. (1990). An integrated theory of the etiology of sexual offending. In W. L. Marshall, D. R. Laws, & H. E. Barbaree (Eds.), *Handbook of sexual assault: Issues, theories, and treatment of the offender* (pp. 257–275). New York, NY: Plenum Press.

McCaw, B., Golding, J. M., Farley, M., & Minkoff, J. R. (2007). Domestic violence and abuse, health status, and social functioning. *Women & Health, 45*(2), 1–23. doi:10.1300/J013v45n02_01

Mountjoy, M., Brackenridge, C., Arrington, M., Blauwet, C., Carska-Sheppard, A., Fasting, K., ... Budgett, R. (2016). International Olympic Committee consensus statement: Harassment and abuse (non-accidental violence) in sport. *British Journal of Sports Medicine, 50*, 1019–1029.

Owton, H., & Sparkes, A. C. (2017). "It stays with you": Multiple evocative representations of dance and future possibilities for studies in sport and physical cultures. *Qualitative Research in Sport, Exercise & Health, 9*, 49–55. doi:10.1080/2159676X.2016.1187662

Owusu-Sekyere, F. & Gervis, M. (2016). In the pursuit of mental toughness: Is creating mentally tough players a disguise for emotional abuse? *International Journal of Coaching Science, 10*(1), 3–23.

Pace, R. (2012, March 3). *Bob Knight: The general's top 20 quotes as a college basketball coach.* Retrieved from https://bleacherreport.com/articles/1080495-bob-knight-the-generals-top-20-quotes-as-a-college-basketball-coach#slide17

Parent, S. (2011). Disclosure of sexual abuse in sport organizations: A case study. *Journal of Child Sexual Abuse, 20*(3), 322–337. doi:10.1080/10538712.2011.573459

Parent, S., & Bannon, J. (2012). Sexual abuse in sport: What about boys? *Children and Youth Services Review, 34*(2), 354–359. doi:10.1016/j.childyouth.2011.11.004

Patricelli, K. (2018). *Why do people abuse?* Retrieved from https://www.mentalhelp.net/articles/why-do-people-abuse/

Reuben, A., Moffitt, T. E., Caspi, A., Belsky, D. W., Harrington, H., Schroeder, F., … Danese, A. (2016), Lest we forget: Comparing retrospective and prospective assessments of adverse childhood experiences in the prediction of adult health. *Journal of Child Psychology and Psychiatry, 57*, 1103–1112. doi:10.1111/jcpp.12621

Sansone, R., Kelley, A., & Forbis, J. (2013). Abuse in childhood and religious/spiritual status in adulthood among internal medicine outpatients. *Journal of Religion and Health, 52*(4), 1085–1092.

Stinson, J. D., Sales, B. D., & Becker, J. V. (2008). *Sex offending: Causal theories to inform research, prevention and treatment.* Washington, DC: American Psychological Association.

Stirling, A. E., & Kerr, G. A. (2008). Defining and categorizing emotional abuse in sport. *European Journal of Sport Science, 8*(4), 173–181, doi:10.1080/17461390802086281

Stirling, A. E., & Kerr, G. A. (2009). Abused athletes' perceptions of the coach–athlete relationship. *Sport in Society, 12*(2), 227–239. doi:10.1080/17430430802591019

Stirling, A. E., & Kerr, G. A. (2013). The perceived effects of elite athletes' experiences of emotional abuse in the coach–athlete relationship. *International Journal of Sport and Exercise Psychology, 11*(1), 87–100. doi:10.1080/1612197X.2013.752173

Straus, M. A., & Field, C. J. (2003). Psychological aggression by American parents: National data on prevalence, chronicity, and severity. *Journal of Marriage and Family, 65.* 795–808. doi:10.1111/j.1741-3737.2003.00795.x

Tracy, N. (2016). *Emotional abuse: Definitions, signs, symptoms, examples.* Retrieved from https://www.healthyplace.com/abuse/emotional-psychological-abuse/emotional-abuse-definitions-signs-symptoms-examples

Tschan, W. (2013). *Professional sexual misconduct in institutions: Causes and consequences, prevention and intervention.* Boston, MA: Hogrefe.

Truman, J. (2011). *National crime victimization survey 2010.* U.S. Department of Justice, Office of Justice Programs, Bureau of Justice Statistics. Retrieved from http://bjs.ojp.usdoj.gov/content/pub/pdf/cv10.pdf

Vasilevski, V., & Tucker, A. (2015). Wide-ranging cognitive deficits in adolescents following early life maltreatment. *Neuropsychology, 30.* 10.1037/neu0000215.

Vertommen, T., Schipper-van, N. H., Hartill, M. J., & Den Eede, F. V. (2015). Sexual harassment and abuse in sport: The NOC*NSF helpline. *International Review for the Sociology of Sport, 50*(7), 822–839. doi:10.1177/1012690213498079

Ward, T., & Keenan, T. (1999). Child molesters' implicit theories. *Journal of Interpersonal Violence, 14*, 821–838.

7

INJURY

Nora is in the midst of a breakout season on an elite travel volleyball club. After years of hard work and improvement, she is finally beginning to get noticed by college coaches, and a scholarship offer seems inevitable. While warming up for a midseason practice, Nora is inadvertently tripped by a teammate and huts her wrist trying to break the fall. Not wanting to seem like a "baby," Nora gets right back up and re-enters drills. Both her teammate and the athletic trainer quickly come over to see that Nora is ok, and despite being in pain, she assures them that she is fine. That night at home Nora's wrist becomes swollen and the pain continues. She makes the decision to play through the pain so as not to lose her opportunity to be seen by college coaches. Unfortunately, her play begins to suffer, and soon her coach demands that she sit out and receive treatment. A scan reveals serious ligament damage, and Nora is told that she will likely miss most of the remaining games. Left without the game that she has devoted years to, the prospect of losing a scholarship opportunity, and isolation from her team while she rehabs, Nora falls into a mild state of depression in the weeks to follow.

Perhaps no other threat to athletes' psychosocial health is as pervasive as physical injury. Any athlete that competes for an extended period is sure to encounter one, and likely multiple, acute and chronic injuries over the course of their career. One need only spend a few days examining sports websites to learn of the many and varied injuries experienced by high-level athletes in all sports. The NCAA and National Athletic Trainers Association report approximately

12,500 injuries requiring athletes to miss at least one day of practice per year since 1982 (Agel, Evans, Dick, Putukian, & Marshall, 2007). In Europe, over 4 million athletes per year over the age of 15 are treated in a hospital for a sport injury (Kisser & Bauer, 2010). Certain sports carry more risk than others. A cursory review of the injury report for week 10 of the 2017 National Football League (NFL) season revealed more than 100 players across 13 games. Sport injuries can range from relatively minor sprains and strains to more serious spinal cord damage and head trauma. And although most injuries do not have a direct effect on athletes' cognitive, emotional, social, or spiritual functioning, the resulting loss of function and process of recovery can challenge all aspects of psychosocial health.

The psychosocial aspects of sport injury have been the subject of more articles, chapters, and books than any of the other threats discussed in this text. I encourage interested readers to consult recent texts by Arvinen-Barrow and Walker (2013) and Brewer and Redmond (2017) for a comprehensive treatment of relevant research and theory. My focus in this chapter is on the psychosocial antecedents and consequences of sport injury for high-level athletes. I begin with a discussion of research and theory related to the psychosocial antecedents of sport injury. This is followed by a general focus on the psychosocial health consequences of sport injury, including a focus on aspects of the rehabilitation recovery process instrumental to athletes' psychosocial functioning. I then address two types of sport injury that warrant special consideration related to athletes' psychosocial health: (a) spinal cord injuries, and (b) concussions. The chapter concludes with recommendations for future research.

Psychosocial antecedents of sport injury

The notion that psychosocial phenomena can influence susceptibility to illness dates to the work of psychiatrists Holmes and Rahe (1967), who established a link between stressful life events such as the death of a spouse, divorce, and retirement and subsequent illness. More recently, the field of psychoneuroimmunology has been established to understand how chronic stress compromises individuals' immune system and leads to disease (e.g., Goodkin & Visser, 2000). In the early 1980s, sport psychology researchers began to wonder whether a similar link existed between life stress and sport injury. Results were equivocal, as some showed a positive relationship between life stress and sport injury (e.g., Cryan & Alles, 1983; Hardy & Riehl, 1988; Passer & Seese, 1983), and some did not (e.g., Passer & Seese, 1983; Williams, Tonymon, & Wadsworth, 1986). As research progressed, other variables, such as personality and social support and coping skills were integrated for a more complete explanation of the psychosocial antecedents of sport injury. Informed by such work, Andersen and Williams (1988) made the first significant theoretical advancement related to the psychosocial pre-cursors of sport injury.

Andersen and Williams' (1988) model of stress and athletic injury

The Model of Stress and Athletic Injury proposed by Andersen and Williams (1988; 1998) remains one of the most influential frameworks in the field of sport psychology. The authors drew from other models of stress in and out of sport, as well as extant life stress and sport injury research in developing the model, which contains three interacting "layers" of psychosocial factors proposed to influence athletes' likelihood of injury: (a) the top layer focusing on factors of the person, including their history of stressors, personality, and coping resources, (b) the middle layer focusing on the process of injury occurrence, including athletes' appraisal of different sport situations and resulting muscular and attentional changes, and (c) the bottom layer focusing on cognitive behavioral interventions that may modify the process described in the middle layer by arming athletes with the skills to more effectively appraise situations and manage their bodily reactions to potentially stressful situations.

For example, consider a basketball player with perfectionistic tendencies (e.g., obsessive focus on results), who faces daily organizational stressors in the form of financial uncertainty and worries about her place on the team, and who lacks effective coping skills (top layer). According to the model, the interacting influence of the athlete's characteristics puts her at risk of appraising stressful basketball situations (e.g., a game against a rival club) as threatening, resulting in excess muscle tension, and perhaps reduced attention for relevant environmental cues during the game (middle layer). However, the effect of the top layer on the middle layer can be moderated by education and training on physical relaxation, focus, and self-talk from a certified mental-performance consultant.

Subsequent research has supported the various components of Andersen and Williams' model, as researchers have employed it to understand the patterns of personality, stressors, and coping most linked to injury (top layer), as well as interventions to help athletes manage their thoughts and arousal (bottom layer) (Williams & Andersen, 1998). Personality characteristics linked to injury include sensation seeking (Smith, Ptacek, & Smoll, 1992), locus of control (Hanson, McCullagh, & Tonymon, 1992), Type A personality (Gill, Henderson, & Pargman, 1995), and hardiness (Chung, 2012). One shortcoming of the model is its questionable applicability to the occurrence of chronic overuse sport injuries that can occur in all sports, but that are particularly prevalent in individual endurance sports such as running and cycling.

The role of the sport ethic in athletic injury

Although Andersen and Williams' (1988) model offers a cogent explanation for acute injuries in high-level sport, some injuries are more effectively explained from a sociological perspective. In Chapter 5 I highlighted the work of sport sociologists Jay Coakley and Michael Messner, who first brought attention to and critiqued implicit norms of high-level sport that pose a risk to athletes' psychosocial and physical health. The four norms of sport proposed by Hughes and Coakley (1991)—making sacrifices for the game, striving for distinction, accepting risks and playing through pain, and refusing to accept limits—are collectively termed the *sport ethic*. Although one can argue that all four norms operate to increase the likelihood of injury for athletes, the third norm is particularly relevant for sport injuries caused by overtraining and/or playing despite injury. Recent research supports a relationship between the sport ethic and athletes' playing through pain and injury. Madrigal, Robbins, Gill, and Wurst (2015) interviewed male and female collegiate rugby players to better understand why they chose to risk further injury by playing while hurt. Many of the athletes' responses aligned with norms of the sport ethic introduced by Hughes and Coakley. Players noted how their decision about whether to play while hurt largely depended on the importance of the contest (i.e., sacrifice), and how their beliefs about playing while hurt were shaped by coaches' mixed message that although they shouldn't play while "injured," they should play while "hurt" (i.e., accepting risks).

The issue of playing through pain and injury has recently garnered mainstream attention due to the recognition of concussions as a serious health threat for athletes. A powerful reminder of the psychosocial pull felt by athletes to play through pain and injury is the perspective of a young field-hockey player who blacked out during a game after being hit in the head with an opponent's stick: "The only thought in my mind was getting back in the game. I thought I had to be tough. I thought I had to go back in because we were losing and I needed to support my team" (Murray, 2014, para. 2). According to Murray (2014), the concussion sustained by the athlete led to months of physical therapy for loss of balance, and the onset of ADHD leading to reduced academic performance. Such an attitude is even more pervasive at the highest levels of sport, where athletes', coaches, and administrators' jobs face intense scrutiny to produce results or risk losing their job. In a story for CNN in 2010, recently retired NFL quarterback Kurt Warner spoke of the culture of high-level sport in which playing while injured is supported, and sitting out is viewed as a sign of weakness.

> There's always a big push from an organization and coaches because obviously that's their livelihood and they want their best players out there playing ... I don't think anybody came up to me and said, "Well you have to play whether you're 100 percent or not, we need you." Nobody said anything like that. But you wondered if guys were looking at you a little differently and saying ... he's not being tough.
>
> (Smith, 2010, para. 3–4)

In addition to the sport ethic, Warner's quote evokes notions of the culture of masculinity which predominates high-level sport, and especially contact sports such as American football. Hegemonic forms of masculinity, such as those found in sport, dictate that "real athletes" are tough, emotionless, and take risks for the team (Fainaru & Fainaru, 2014). Of course, as discussed in Chapter 5, and as seen in the aforementioned study by Madrigal et al. (2015), high-level female athletes can also fall prey to the rules of hegemonic masculinity.

Summary

Whereas Andersen and Williams' (1988) model provides a viable explanation for the psychosocial antecedents of acute injuries in sport, Hughes and Coakley's (1991) concept of the sport ethic seems to better account for sport injuries attributable to overtraining and playing through pain. Both explanations offer support for the role of cognitive, emotional, and social factors in placing high-level athletes at risk for sport injury. Thus, although there is no substitute for proper and preventive physical strengthening and conditioning, research suggests that a truly comprehensive injury prevention program addresses the psychosocial precursors to injury as well.

Psychosocial consequences of sport injury

The more severe an injury to an athlete's body, the greater the implications for psychosocial health. Common negative psychosocial consequences of injury include loss of identity (Lockhart, 2010), fears associated with missing time and/or returning to play (Kvist, 2005), and social isolation (Gould, Udry, Bridges, & Beck, 1997). Since the 1990's, several theories and many studies have been devoted to understanding and explaining the influence of sport injury on athletes' subsequent thoughts, emotions, relationships, and behaviors (e.g., Hardy & Crace, 1990; Gould et al., 1997; Petitpas & Danish, 1995; Podlog & Eklund, 2006; Wiese-Bjornstal, Smith, Shaffer, & Morrey, 1998).

Hardy and Crace (1990) suggested a parallel between athletes' process of dealing with an injury and the process of grieving the death of a loved one proposed by Kübler-Ross (1969). From the perspective of the stages of grief, athletes navigate through a predictable pattern of thoughts, emotions, and behaviors post-injury, including denial, anger, bargaining, depression, and acceptance. Although the stage approach to explaining athletes' psychosocial response to injury makes intuitive sense, and has garnered some research support (e.g., Gordon, Milios, & Grove, 1991), it has been largely rejected as overly restrictive and not necessarily consistent with the experience of all athletes (Gould et al., 1997). However, one element of Kübler-Ross' model not often discussed in connection with sport injury, is the spiritual implication of the bargaining stage, in which athletes are said to negotiate with a higher power for a return to normalcy or even for the injury itself to have never happened. Despite acknowledgment from professionals on the relevance of spirituality/religion for athletes' rehabilitation (e.g., McKnight & Juillerat, 2011), surprisingly little research has focused on the spiritual domain of health. It would be interesting to examine whether spiritual health can buffer athletes from negative post-injury outcomes relative to other domains of psychosocial health, or how spiritual health itself is directly affected by injury.

In the late 1990s, Wiese-Bjornstal et al. (1998) proposed a sport-specific model to explain athletes' emotional and behavioral responses to sport injury. Drawing from previous research and theory on the psychology of sport injury, the authors portrayed athletes' sport injury responses occurring in the context of personal factors (e.g., injury history, personality, ethnicity, overall physical health) and situational factors (e.g., sport type, sport ethic, rehabilitation environment). According to the model, the influence of personal and situational factors on responses to injury is mediated by athletes' cognitive appraisal, which includes self-perceptions, attributions, and self-efficacy. Athletes' appraisal sets the stage for emotional responses such as fear, frustration, boredom, or depression. Wiese-Bjornstal et al. are careful to highlight the fact that the majority of injured athletes have a positive attitude and cope well with injury. Further, they call into question the assumption that negative emotions are inherently "bad," as such emotions may serve to motivate athletes toward recovery. A strength of the integrated model is its recognition of the various components as interdependent, and athletes' responses and associated recovery outcomes as ever-changing. Research supports the dynamic nature of athletes' response to injury, as cognitive appraisals, coping strategies, and even psychological characteristics evolve from pre-injury until return to play (e.g., Clement , Arvinen-Barrow, & Fetty, 2015; Madrigal & Gill, 2014).

Acknowledging the complex and dynamic nature of response to injury and rehabilitation, Brewer, Andersen, and Van Raalte (2002) proposed a biopsychosocial model to specifically explain athletes' return to sport experience. The model contains a litany of interdependent biological, psychological, and social factors and sub-factors suggested to influence athletes' return to sport outcomes. To start the process, characteristics of the injury (e.g., severity) combine with sociodemographic characteristics of athletes (e.g., age) to influence biological (e.g., tissue repair), psychological (e.g., cognition), and social (e.g., social support) responses. These three factors interact to influence intermediate outcomes such as rate of recovery, and long-term rehabilitation outcomes such as treatment satisfaction (Brewer et al., 2002). Although the biopsychosocial model offers a broad framework for the study of return to play, Podlog and Eklund (2007) contend that it does not offer the specificity necessary to explain different return to sport outcomes.

Other researchers have adopted more mainstream theories of motivation and behavior to understand athletes' psychosocial responses to injury, and the environmental factors that contribute to these responses. As one of the predominant theories used to understand and explain behavior in sport, self-determination theory (SDT) has proven useful in this regard. Although comprised of several sub-theories, the basic premise of Deci and Ryan's (1985) SDT is that individuals' motivation for a given behavior ranges on a continuum from amotivation (i.e., not at all motivated) to intrinsic motivation (i.e., engaging in the behavior for the sheer satisfaction of doing it). SDT posits that the more an individual experiences satisfaction of the three basic psychosocial needs of competence, autonomy, and relatedness, the more intrinsic their motivation. Because more self-determined motivation is associated with higher performance, persistence, creativity, and well-being (Ryan & Deci, 2000), a large body of research in sport has focused on how sport environments can support or thwart athletes' psychosocial needs, and the subsequent psychosocial outcomes (e.g., Mallett & Hanrahan, 2004; Sheldon & Watson, 2011).

Within the realm of sport injury, Podlog et al. (Podlog & Eklund, 2005; Podlog & Eklund, 2006; Podlog & Eklund, 2007; Podlog & Eklund, 2009; Podlog & Eklund, 2010; Podlog, Lochbaum, & Stevens, 2010) have been at the forefront of work establishing links between components of SDT and return to sport outcomes in injured athletes. In sum, the extent to which high-level athletes perceive positive psychological outcomes from their injury such as a renewed perspective seems at least partially dependent on how intrinsically motivated they are to return to play (Podlog & Eklund, 2005). Issues of competency, autonomy, and relatedness may underlie common emotional responses to injury such as fear, isolation, and loss of identity (Podlog & Eklund, 2007; Podlog & Eklund, 2009).

Studies support the importance of a need-fulfilling motivational climate for athletes' return to sport experience. For example, hints of the three needs of competence, autonomy, and relatedness were evident in the responses of formerly injured high-level athletes interviewed by Podlog and Eklund (2009) for a study on perceptions of success in return to sport. In terms of competence, several athletes gauged their return as successful because they overcame adversity. One athlete said, "I think it's a test of your character and a test of your will and determination to get back to where you want to be" (Podlog & Eklund, 2009, p. 541). The influence of autonomy was shown as athletes discussed perceived pressure from parents and coaches to not only return within a certain timeframe, but successfully achieve performance goals upon their return. Finally, the importance of relatedness was evident as athletes discussed helpful coach feedback and involvement with the team as central to a successful return. As one athlete voiced, encouragement from his coach not only contributed to a sense of competence, but relatedness as well: "the coach was pretty happy with my performances and he indicated it to me verbally so that's the greatest indication I have [of my return-to-sport success]" (Podlog & Eklund, 2009, p. 540). Thus, satisfaction of the three psychosocial needs of competence, autonomy, and relatedness appear critical in shaping athletes' emotional responses to injury and perceptions of the recovery process. When needs are met, athletes are not only more motivated to return, but more satisfied with their return as well.

Summary

A multitude of theories and models have been put forth to explain the psychosocial consequences of sport injury. Early frameworks supporting a linear stage-like progression of relevant psychosocial responses from injury to return have been replaced by multifactor models emphasizing the fluidity of athletes' response depending on biological, psychological, and social factors. SDT has emerged as a useful theory for understanding the mechanisms underlying athletes' emotional responses to injury and rehabilitation. It seems that optimal psychosocial outcomes are more likely to occur when athletes' psychosocial needs are met throughout the process of recovery.

Spinal cord injuries and concussions

Because of their career-ending and life-altering potential, injuries affecting the central nervous system (i.e., brain and spinal cord) are among those with the greatest implications for athletes' psychosocial health. Because so little research has examined the psychosocial health consequences of sport-based SCI and concussions in athletes of any kind (whether high-level or recreational), I include studies with athletes at any level of participation to illustrate the psychosocial impact of these injuries.

According to the National Spinal Cord Injury Statistical Center (NSCISC, 2016), of the approximately 282,000 Americans who suffered a spinal cord injury (SCI) in 2016, more than 25,000 occurred in the act of a sport or recreational activity. In countries such as Russia and Canada, sport participation accounts for more than 13% of SCIs. Whereas SCIs affecting the cervical vertebrae are the most common type in collision sports such as American football and speed sports such as downhill skiing, thoracic and lumbosacral injuries are more common in horseback riding and snowboarding (Chan, Eng, Tator, & Krassioukov, 2016). Depending on the severity, symptoms of SCIs range from numbness, to loss of muscle function, to paralysis. Whereas *incomplete* injuries result in partial loss of motor function below the injury site, *complete* injuries result in total loss of function. In the most extreme case, a complete SCI occurring to the upper cervical vertebrae results in loss of autonomous ventilatory function, and the end of an athlete's career (Sabharwal, 2013). Although such injuries are rare, former Rutgers University American football player Eric LeGrand fractured his C3 and C4 vertebrae during a collision during a 2010 game. Although LeGrand has since regained some use of his upper body, he still requires a wheelchair (Politi, 2018).

In one of the earlier studies on SCI in sport, Smith and Sparkes (2005) engaged in in-depth narrative analysis of interviews with 14 men who sustained injuries leading to paralysis while playing rugby. The authors were specifically interested in how these men talked about hope, and it was found that the men conceptualized hope in one of three ways: (a) concrete hope (e.g., hope of finding a cure), (b) transcendent hope (e.g., hope of gaining something valuable from the SCI experience), and (c) despair (e.g., things will never get better). Later, Smith (2013) used a storytelling approach to represent the views of 20 men in rehabilitation from an SCI sustained while playing sport. The central finding of Smith's novel study was how the psychosocial consequences of sport-based SCI were neither solely dependent on athletes' social environment (e.g., social structures, views of others) nor their personal attributes, but rather they were the product of dynamic interactions between people with SCI and their social environment (i.e., social relations). That is, past and anticipated future social interactions shape how people with an SCI think, feel, and act.

Much more common than SCI in sport are traumatic brain injuries (TBI) due to sport-related concussions (SRCs). As compared to SCIs, the damage caused by SRCs is often invisible, and may not truly be revealed until years after the initial injury. The Centers for Disease Control and Prevention define concussions as:

> a type of traumatic brain injury … caused by a bump, blow, or jolt to the head or by a hit to the body that causes the head and brain to move rapidly back and forth. This sudden movement can cause the brain to bounce around or twist in the skull, creating chemical changes in the brain and sometimes stretching and damaging brain cells.
>
> *(Centers for Disease Control and Prevention, 2017, para. 1)*

According to a five-year epidemiologic study sponsored by the NCAA, there were 1,670 SRCs in NCAA athletes between 2009 and 2014, corresponding to a rate of 4.47 SRCs per 10,000 athlete-practices or competitions (Zuckerman, Kerr, Yengo-Kahn, Wasserman, Covassin, & Solomon, 2015). SRCs are particularly common in collision sports such as American football, boxing, and ice hockey, but also often occur in soccer, lacrosse, and water polo (Blumenfeld, Winsell, Hicks, & Small, 2016; Förstl, Haass, Hemmer, Meyer, & Halle, 2010; Zuckerman et al., 2015). Although boxing is by far the deadliest sport—an average of 10 deaths per year since 1890 (Förstl et al., 2010)—the extreme popularity of American football in the U.S. means that it has been the subject of most media attention and scholarly research on SRCs.

Once treated as a natural part of contact sports (e.g., "He's ok, he just had his bell rung a bit."), a rash of reported cognitive impairments to and suicides of former American football players in the last ten years has raised awareness of the potential danger of high-impact collisions, as well as accumulated low-impact blows to the head (Breedlove et al., 2012). Of all the threats to athletes' psychosocial health discussed in this text, SRCs undoubtedly pose the largest threat to the cognitive domain. Breedlove et al. (2012) reported the findings of a two-year study of high-school American football players, in which concussions were found to occur because of repeated low-impact blows to the head rather than a single high-impact blow. Further, debilitative changes to the brain were found in several players who did not sustain an SRC over the two seasons. Such changes to athletes' brains may trigger emotional health issues such as anxiety, depression, and suicidal behavior (Covassin, Elbin, Beidler, LaFevor, & Kontos, 2017).

Of greatest concern for the cognitive health of athletes who have sustained one or more SRCs in their career is the potential development of chronic traumatic encephalopathy (CTE)—a neurodegenerative condition characterized by the buildup of protein which disables neuropathways in the brain (Emanuel, 2017). The brain damage caused by CTE can manifest in a variety of negative cognitive and emotional symptoms, including memory loss, confusion, impaired judgment, aggression, depression, anxiety, impulse control, and suicidal behavior (McKee et al., 2009). Research conducted by faculty of Boston University's CTE Center reveals the pervasive nature of CTE for American football players. Of the 202 brains of deceased pre-high-school, high-school, collegiate, and professional American football players examined, 87% showed signs of CTE, including 99% of former NFL players (Mez et al., 2017).

Despite compelling research findings, efforts to prevent serious head injuries and long-term health consequences are hindered by the aforementioned sport ethic, which compels athletes to withhold concussion symptoms for fear that they may lose playing time, or worse, be viewed as lacking toughness. Indeed, many high-level athletes from both high- and low-contact sports continue to subscribe to the notion that concussions are part of what they agreed to when they chose to play their sport, and report intentionally withholding concussion symptoms to preserve their spot on the team (Beverly et al., 2018). Additionally, athletes in low-contact sports such as tennis and swimming may fail to report concussion symptoms out of embarrassment for their "clumsy" actions (Beverly et al., 2018).

Although the risk of TBI associated with contact sports has been acknowledged for several years, it was not until recently that the psychosocial elements of these injuries were examined. Of note is a 2017 special issue of the journal *Sport, Exercise, and Performance Psychology* (SEPP) focused on the psychology of SRCs, in which both pre- and post-psychosocial aspects of SRCs were the subject of investigation. One of the studies in the special issue detailed the predictive utility of several psychosocial variables (e.g., athletic identity, performance anxiety, and motivation) on self-reported symptomatology from 7 to 28 days post-concussion in youth athletes (O'Rourke, Smith, Punt, Coppel, & Breiger, 2017). In brief, lower motivation, higher athletic identity, and higher performance anxiety predicted slower declines in self-reported symptomatology. The authors proposed several underlying mechanisms to explain these findings, including less productive cognitive appraisals of injury from athletes with high athletic identity, less incentive to minimize symptoms for amotivated athletes, and heightened symptom sensitivity in athletes with more performance anxiety.

Several other studies in the special issue of SEPP focused on the psychosocial aftermath of SRCs. Of note is a piece by André-Morin, Caron, & Bloom (2017), which addresses a gap in SRC research by exploring the experiences of collegiate female athletes with protracted concussion symptoms. The authors argue that because contact sports such as American football, in which most participants are men, have been the focus of most SRC research, the experiences of female athletes with SRC have been ignored. The athletes in their study spoke about a number of psychosocial ramifications of their SRC, including depression, mood swings, and social isolation (André-Morin et al.). One athlete said,

"All the things that I knew would usually make me happy and put a smile on my face didn't work" (André-Morin et al., p. 296). One athlete in the study even reported that she attempted suicide. Clearly, male athletes are not alone in dealing with the harmful psychosocial effects of SRCs. And because female athletes may actually experience concussions at a higher rate than male athletes (Covassin, Moran, & Elbin, 2016), further discussion on the potential long-term effects of these injuries for women is warranted.

A final study from the special issue warrants consideration, as it addresses the question of whether the psychosocial responses associated with SRCs are unique in comparison to other common sport injuries. Prompted by previous studies suggesting differences in the psychological responses of athletes with musculo-skeletal versus athletes with an SRC (e.g., Mainwaring, Hutchison, Bisschop, Comper, & Richards, 2010), Turner, Langdon, Shaver, Graham, Naugle, & Buckley, 2017) compared changes in mood and anxiety from up to 72 hours post-injury to return to play in two matched groups of athletes diagnosed with either an SRC (n = 15) or a minor musculoskeletal injury (n = 15). In contrast to the findings of Mainwaring et al. (2010), the authors found no significant difference between the two groups across time in mood or anxiety. Because past studies failed to control for time loss and duration of rehabilitation, the authors concluded that it may be these factors that accounted for disparate psychological responses rather than any physiological changes associated with SRCs.

Summary

SCIs and SRCs are serious injuries to the central nervous system that can end athletes' careers and result in permanent cognitive and/or motor impairments. As such, these injuries may have a particularly profound effect on athletes' cognitive, emotional, social, and spiritual health. Research by Smith on sport-related SCIs shows the variety of ways that athletes negotiate their new reality and possible future, and how their disability experience is the product of dynamic social relations. The more extensive research on SRCs highlights psychosocial influences that may prevent athletes from reporting symptoms, how psychosocial factors influence the cessation of symptomatology, and the wide-ranging cognitive, emotional, and social health implications of SRCs.

Future research directions

Although hundreds of research articles on the psychology of sport injury have been written, more work remains to more clearly understand the consequences of injury for athletes' short- and long-term psychosocial health. Because several theories and models of psychosocial response to sport injury have been proposed (e.g., cognitive appraisal, motivational), it behooves researchers to determine which one best accounts for variations in process and outcome for recovering high-level athletes. SDT seems to offer a promising framework from which to understand athletes' experience of recovery and associated psychosocial health outcomes. Researchers may wish to examine a blending of the cognitive appraisal and SDT approaches, such that psychosocial need satisfaction promotes certain appraisals and subsequent psychosocial health outcomes. Regardless of the theoretical perspective adopted, longitudinal prospective designs with varied samples of athletes and various types of injuries are critical for understanding the pattern of variables influencing psychosocial health outcomes for injured athletes. Mixed-methods studies combining frequent quantitative data collection with qualitative data across the course of injury may also be useful for theory development.

As with most of the other threats discussed in this text, the spiritual dimension of health has been neglected in sport injury research. It might be interesting to explore changes in spiritual health for athletes who have experienced severe SCIs or SRCs, as these injuries pose the greatest risk of long-term physical and cognitive impairment. As discussed further in Chapter 11, serious injuries may even trigger *enhanced* spiritual health. Regardless of the direction of change, there is a need for more studies of sport injury in which spiritual health is a central variable of interest.

Conclusion

Because the focus of media coverage on athlete injury is usually on visible physical health aspects affecting return to play, invisible psychosocial health factors are less discussed. This is unfortunate, as depending on the nature and severity of the injury, athletes' psychosocial health can be equally affected. Extant theories illustrate the multifaceted and dynamic nature of recovery, with most theories emphasizing the influence that relevant personal and situational factors have on athletes' ever-changing appraisals and emotional responses. The SDT is a more recent addition to sport injury research, and holds promise for informing the development of motivational sport climates that buffer athletes from negative psychosocial health outcomes. Although all injuries can potentially affect psychosocial health, SCIs and SRCs are of particular interest due to their impact on athletes' ability to move and think effectively.

References

Agel, J., Evans, T. A., Dick, R., Putukian, M., & Marshall, S. W. (2007). Descriptive epidemiology of collegiate men's soccer injuries: National Collegiate Athletic Association Injury Surveillance System, 1988–1989 through 2002–2003. *Journal of Athletic Training, 42*(2), 270–247.

Andersen, M. B., & Williams, J. M. (1988). A model of stress and athletic injury: Prediction and prevention. *Journal of Sport and Exercise Psychology, 10*(3), 294–306. doi:10.1123/jsep.10.3.294

André-Morin, D., Caron, J. G., & Bloom, G. A. (2017). Exploring the unique challenges faced by female university athletes experiencing prolonged concussion symptoms. *Sport, Exercise, and Performance Psychology, 6*(3), 289–303. doi:10.1037/spy0000106

Arvinen-Barrow, M., & Walker, N. (Eds.). (2013). *The psychology of sport injury and rehabilitation*. Abingdon, United Kingdom: Routledge.

Beverly, E. A., Fredricks, T. R., Leubitz, A., Oldach, B. R., Kana, D., Grant, M. D., ... Guseman, E. H. (2018). What can family medicine providers learn about concussion non-disclosure from former collegiate athletes? *BMC Family Practice, 19*, 128. doi:10.1186/s12875-018-0818-2.

Blumenfeld, R. S., Winsell, J. C., Hicks, J. W., & Small, S. L. (2016). The epidemiology of sports-related head injury and concussion in water polo. *Frontiers in Neurology, 7*, 98. doi:10.3389/fneur.2016.00098

Breedlove, E. L., Robinson, M., Talavage, T. M., Morigaki, K. E., Yoruk, U., O'Keefe, K., ... Nauman, E. A. (2012). Biomechanical correlates of symptomatic and asymptomatic neurophysiological impairment in high school football. *Journal of Biomechanics, 45*, 1265–1272. doi:10.1016/j.jbiomech.2012.01.034.

Brewer, B., & Redmond, C. (2017). Psychology of sport injury. Champaign, IL: Human Kinetics.

Brewer, B. W., Andersen, M. B., & Van Raalte, J. L. (2002). Psychological aspects of sport injury rehabilitation: Toward a biopsychosocial approach. In D. L. Mostofsky (Ed.), *Medical and psychological aspects of sport and exercise* (pp. 41–54). Morgantown, WV: Fitness Information Technology.

Centers for Disease Control and Prevention. (2017). *What is a concussion?* Retrieved from https://www.cdc.gov/headsup/basics/concussion_whatis.html

Chan, C. W. L., Eng, J. J., Tator, C. H., Krassioukov, A., & the Spinal Cord Research Evidence Team. (2016). Epidemiology of sport-related spinal cord injuries: A systematic review. *The Journal of Spinal Cord Medicine, 39*(3), 255–264. doi:10.1080/1 0790268.2016.1138601

Chung, Y. (2012). Psychological correlates of athletic injuries: Hardiness, life stress, and cognitive appraisal. *International Journal of Applied Sports Sciences, 24*(2), 89–98.

Clement, D., Arvinen-Barrow, M., & Fetty, T. (2015). Psychosocial responses during different phases of sport-injury rehabilitation: A qualitative study. *Journal of Athletic Training, 50*(1), 95–104. doi:10.4085/1062-6050-49.3.52

Covassin, T., Elbin, R. J., Beidler, E., LaFevor, M., & Kontos, A. P. (2017). A review of psychological issues that may be associated with a sport-related concussion in youth and collegiate athletes. *Sport, Exercise, and Performance Psychology, 6*(3), 220–229. doi:10.1037/spy0000105

Covassin, T., Moran, R., & Elbin, R. J. (2016). Sex differences in reported concussion injury rates and time loss from participation: An update of the National Collegiate Athletic Association Injury Surveillance Program from 2004–2005 through 2008–2009. *Journal of Athletic Training, 51*(3), 189–194. doi:10.4085/1062-6050-51.3.05

Cryan, P. D., & Alles, W. F. (1983). The relationship between stress and college football injuries. *Journal of Sports Medicine & Physical Fitness, 23*(1), 52–58.

Deci, E., & Ryan, R. M. (1985). *Intrinsic motivation and self-determination in human behavior*. New York, NY: Plenum Press.

Emanuel, D. (2017, July 26). *CTE found in 99% of studied brains from deceased NFL players*. Retrieved from https://www.cnn.com/2017/07/25/health/cte-nfl-players-brains-study/index.html

Fainaru-Wada, M., & Fainaru, S. (2014). *League of denial: The NFL, concussions, and the battle for truth*. New York, NY: Three Rivers Press.

Förstl, H., Haass, C., Hemmer, B., Meyer, B., & Halle, M. (2010). Boxing-acute complications and late sequelae: From concussion to dementia. *Deutsches Arzteblatt International, 107*(47), 835–839. doi:10.3238/arztebl.2010.0835

Gill, K., Henderson, J., & Pargman, D. (1995). The type A competitive runner: at risk for psychological stress and injury? *International Journal of Sport Psychology, 26*(4), 541–550.

Goodkin. K., & Visser, A. P. (Eds.). (2000). *Psychoneuroimmunology: Stress, mental disorders, and health.* Washington, DC: American Psychiatric Association.

Gordon, S., Milios, D., & Grove, J. R. (1991). Psychological aspects of the recovery process from sport injury: The perspective of sport physiotherapists. *Australian Journal of Science & Medicine in Sport, 23*(2), 53–60.

Gould, D., Udry, E., Bridges, D., & Beck. (1997). How to help elite athletes cope psychologically with season-ending injuries. *Athletic Therapy Today, 2*(4), 50–53.

Hanson, S. J., McCullagh, P., & Tonymon, P. (1992). The relationship of personality characteristics, life stress, and coping resources to athletic injury. *Journal of Sport and Exercise Psychology, 14*(3), 262–272. doi:10.1123/jsep.14.3.262

Hardy, C. J., & Crace, R. K. (1990). *Dealing with injury. Sport Psychology Training Bulletin, 1,* 1–8.

Hardy, C. J., & Riehl, R. E. (1988). An examination of the life stress–injury relationship among noncontact sport participants. *Behavioral Medicine, 14*(3), 113–118. doi:10.108 0/08964289.1988.9935132

Holmes, T. H., & Rahe, R. H. (1967). The Social Readjustment Rating Scale. *Journal of Psychosomatic Research, 11*(2), 213–218. doi:10.1016/0022-3999(67)90010-4

Hughes, R., & Coakley, J. (1991). Positive deviance among athletes: The implications of overconformity to the sport ethic. *Sociology of Sport Journal, 8,* 307–325. doi:10.1123/ssj.8.4.307

Kisser, R., & Bauer, R. (2010). Sport injuries in the European Union. *Injury Prevention, 16,* A211.

Kübler-Ross, E. (1969). *On death and dying.* New York, NY: Macmillan.

Kvist, J., Ek, A., Sporrstedt, K., & Good, L. (2005). Fear of re-injury: A hindrance for returning to sports after anterior cruciate ligament reconstruction. *Knee Surgery, Sports Traumatology, Arthroscopy, 13*(5), 393–397. Retrieved from https://doi.org/10.1007/s00167-004-0591-8

Lockhart, B. D. (2010). Injured athletes' perceived loss of identity: Educational implications for athletic trainers. *Athletic Training Education Journal, 5*(1), 26–31.

Madrigal, L., & Gill, D. L. (2014). Psychological responses of Division I female athletes throughout injury recovery: A case study approach. *Journal of Clinical Sport Psychology, 8*(3), 276–298. doi:10.1123/jcsp.2014-0034

Madrigal, L., Robbins, J., Gill, D. L., & Wurst, K. (2015). A pilot study investigating the reasons for playing through pain and injury: Emerging themes in men's and women's collegiate rugby. *The Sport Psychologist, 29*(4), 310–318. doi:10.1123/tsp.2014-0139

Mainwaring, L. M., Hutchison, M., Bisschop, S. M., Comper, P., & Richards, D. W. (2010). Emotional response to sport concussion compared to ACL injury. *Brain Injury, 24*(4), 589–597. doi:10.3109/02699051003610508

Mallett, C. J., & Hanrahan, S. J. (2004). Elite athletes: Why does the "fire" burn so brightly? *Psychology of Sport and Exercise, 5*(2), 183–200. doi:10.1016/S1469-0292(02)00043-2.

McKee, A. C., Cantu, R. C., Nowinski, C. J., Hedley-Whyte, E. T., Gavett, B. E., Budson, A. E., ... Stern, R. A. (2009). Chronic traumatic encephalopathy in athletes: Progressive tauopathy after repetitive head injury. *Journal of Neuropathology & Experimental Neurology, 68,* 709–735. doi:10.1097/NEN.0b013e3181a9d503

McKnight, C. M., & Juillerat, S. (2011). Perceptions of clinical athletic trainers on the spiritual care of injured athletes. *Journal of Athletic Training, 46*(3), 303–311. doi:10.4085/1062-6050-46.3.303

Mez, J., Daneshvar, D. H., Kiernan, P. T., Abdolmohammadi, B., Alvarez, V. E., Huber, B. R., ... McKee, A. C. (2017). Clinicopathological evaluation of chronic traumatic encephalopathy in players of American football. *JAMA, 318*(4), 360–370. doi:10.1001/jama.2017.8334

Murray, E. (2014, November 8). *Teens playing through pain, not taking sports injuries seriously, says study.* Retrieved from https://www.today.com/health/teens-playing-through-pain-not-taking-sports-injuries-seriously-says-1D80274256

National Spinal Cord Injury Statistical Center. (2016). *Spinal cord injury (SCI): Facts and figures at a glance.* Retrieved from https://www.nscisc.uab.edu/Public/Facts%20 2016.pdf

O'Rourke, D. J., Smith, R. E., Punt, S., Coppel, D. B., & Breiger, D. (2017). Psychosocial correlates of young athletes' self-reported concussion symptoms during the course of recovery. *Sport, Exercise, and Performance Psychology, 6*(3), 262–276.

Passer, M. W., & Seese, M. D. (1983). Life stress and athletic injury: Examination of positive versus negative events and three moderator variables. *Journal of Human Stress, 9*(4), 11–16. doi:10.1080/0097840X.1983.9935025

Petitpas, A., & Danish, S. J. (1995). Caring for injured athletes. In S. M. Murphy (Ed.), *Sport psychology interventions* (pp. 255–281). Champaign, IL: Human Kinetics.

Podlog, L., & Eklund, R. C. (2005). Return to sport after serious injury: A retrospective examination of motivation and psychological outcomes. *Journal of Sport rehabilitation, 14*(1), 20–34. doi:10.1123/jsr.14.1.20

Podlog, L., & Eklund, R. C. (2006). A longitudinal investigation of competitive athletes' return to sport following serious injury. *Journal of Applied Sport Psychology, 18*(1), 44–68. doi:10.1080/10413200500471319

Podlog, L., & Eklund, R. C. (2007). The psychosocial aspects of a return to sport following serious injury: A review of the literature from a self-determination perspective. *Psychology of Sport and Exercise, 8*(4), 535–566. doi:10.1016/j.psychsport.2006.07.008

Podlog, L., & Eklund, R. C. (2009). High-level athletes' perceptions of success in returning to sport following injury. *Psychology of Sport and Exercise, 10*(5), 535–544. doi:10.1016/j.psychsport.2009.02.003

Podlog, L., & Eklund, R. C. (2010). Returning to competition after a serious injury: The role of self-determination, *Journal of Sports Sciences, 28*(8), 819–831. doi:10.1080/02640411003792729

Podlog, L., Lochbaum, M., & Stevens, T. (2010). Need satisfaction, well-being, and perceived return-to-sport outcomes among injured athletes. *Journal of Applied Sport Psychology, 22*(2), 167–182. doi:10.1080/10413201003664665

Politi, S. (2018, July 30). *The Eric LeGrand you haven't seen ... his private struggle ... in moments away from the spotlight.* Retrieved from https://projects.nj.com/investigations/legrand/

Ryan, R. M., & Deci, E. L. (2000). Intrinsic and extrinsic motivations: Classic definitions and new directions. *Contemporary Educational Psychology, 25*(1), 54–67. doi:10.1006/ceps.1999.1020

Sabharwal, S. (2013). *Essentials of spinal cord medicine.* New York, NY: Demos Medical.

Sheldon, K. M., & Watson, A. (2011). Coach's autonomy support is especially important for varsity compared to club and recreational athletes. *International Journal of Sports Science & Coaching, 6*(1), 109–123. doi:10.1260/1747-9541.6.1.109

Smith, B. (2013). Sporting spinal cord injuries, social relations, and rehabilitation narratives: An ethnographic creative non-fiction of becoming disabled through sport. *Sociology of Sport Journal, 30*, 132–152. doi:10.1123/ssj.30.2.132

Smith, B., & Sparkes, A. C. (2005). Men, sport, spinal cord injury, and narratives of hope. *Social Science & Medicine, 61,* 1095–1105. doi:10.1016/j.socscimed.2005.01.011

Smith, R. E., Ptacek, J. T., & Smoll, F. L. (1992). Sensation seeking, stress, and adolescent injuries: A test of stress-buffering, risk-taking, and coping skills hypotheses. *Journal of Personality and Social Psychology, 62,* 1016–1024. doi:10.1037/0022-3514.62.6.1016

Smith, S. (2010, November 22). Warner: Playing through concussion "part of the game". *CNN Medical News.* Retrieved from http://www.cnn.com/2010/HEALTH/11/22/ playing.through.concussions/index.html

Turner, S., Langdon, J., Shaver, G., Graham, V., Naugle, K., & Buckley, T. (2017). Comparison of psychological response between concussion and musculoskeletal injury in collegiate athletes. *Sport, Exercise, and Performance Psychology, 6*(3), 277–288. doi:10.1037/spy0000099

Wiese-bjornstal, D. M., Smith, A. M., Shaffer, S. M., & Morrey, M. A. (1998). An integrated model of response to sport injury: Psychological and sociological dynamics. *Journal of Applied Sport Psychology, 10*(1), 46–69. doi:10.1080/10413209808406377

Williams, J. M., & Andersen, M. B. (1998). Psychosocial antecedents of sport injury: Review and critique of the stress and injury model. *Journal of Applied Sport Psychology, 10*(1), 5–25. doi:10.1080/10413209808406375

Williams, J. M., Tonymon, P., & Wadsworth, W. A. (1986). Relationship of life stress to injury in intercollegiate volleyball. *Journal of Human Stress, 12*(1), 38–43. doi:10.1080 /0097840X.1986.9936765

Zuckerman, S. L., Kerr, Z. Y., Yengo-Kahn, A., Wasserman, E., Covassin, T., & Solomon, G. S. (2015). Epidemiology of sports-related concussion in NCAA athletes from 2009–2010 to 2013–2014: Incidence, recurrence, and mechanisms. *The American Journal of Sports Medicine, 43*(11), 2654–2662. doi:10.1177/0363546515599634

8

TRANSITIONS

Joaquin is a freshman on a high-level college swim team. In high school, he was the top swimmer on his team, and consistently won or placed in local and regional meets. His swimming accolades earned him much respect and adulation among his teammates and non-swimming friends. Based on his high-school accomplishments, Joaquin was highly recruited by several top universities, and he was excited to earn a partial scholarship to swim at the collegiate level. Unfortunately, things have not gone as he envisioned. First, he is no longer the top swimmer on his team, and is fighting to even have a spot at meets. Second, he is struggling to fit in among his teammates, as the older swimmers all hang out together, and there is a competitive atmosphere among the other freshmen that prevents social bonding. Finally, Joaquin is homesick, and has recently found himself wanting nothing more than to quit the team and transfer to the community college 300 miles away, near his family.

In sport, as in life, change is inevitable. Whether, as with Joaquin, it be to a higher level of competition with a new team, or other common sport transitions, such as a new sport, a new country, or retirement, successful athletes are frequently challenged to smoothly transition to new sport and life circumstances. In the strictest sense, *transition* refers to the process or period of change from one state or condition to another (transition, 2018). In the context of human functioning, transitions are planned or unplanned life-altering events that cause people to re-evaluate their sense of self and assumptions about the world (Janoff-Bulman, 2002; Parkes, 1971; Schlossberg, 1981). Within sport, a transition is "a turning phase in athletes' development that brings a set of demands and requires adequate coping processes in order to continue athletic and parallel careers, such as education or work" (Stambulova, 2017, p. 62).

As opposed to some of the other threats to athlete psychosocial health discussed in this text, such as abuse, transitions are not inherently debilitative. For example, although a promotion from an amateur to a professional rugby club may certainly be stressful due to increased time demands and the introduction of performance-contingent financial rewards, it is equally likely to induce positive emotions such as pride, excitement, and nervous anticipation. Furthermore, such transitions are integral for personal growth and development (Leikas & Salmela-Aro, 2014). Nonetheless, athletes who are ill-prepared for or not properly supported during major sport transitions risk missing out on the psychosocial health benefits of transition, or worse, harm to their psychosocial health.

In this chapter I address the potential threat to athlete psychosocial health posed by sport-related transitions. Using the influential work of Nancy Schlossberg (1981) as a guide, I begin with an overview of key concepts related to life transition in adults. Largely informed by the work of Wylleman et al. (e.g., Wylleman, Alfermann, & Lavallee, 2004) and Stambulova et al. (e.g., Franck & Stambulova, 2017), I continue with a discussion of sport-specific perspectives on transition and athlete psychosocial health, including both the transition out of sport as well as within-sport transitions. Finally, I conclude with suggestions for further research to advance our understanding of transition and psychosocial health in athletes.

Foundations of transition

Arguably the most influential general model of life transition in adults is Nancy Schlossberg's (1981) Model of Human Adaptation to Transition. Heavily influenced by theories of adult development, Schlossberg's seminal article laid the groundwork for the study of life transitions by operationally defining the broad types of transitions experienced by adults, and identifying the factors determining how individuals' succeed in managing life transitions. First, Schlossberg posited that most life transitions can be conceptualized as (a) anticipated (e.g., choosing to begin graduate school), (b) unanticipated (e.g., an unexpected job transfer) or (c) non-events (e.g., not receiving an expected pay raise). For a high-level athlete, an anticipated transition might be the completion of their collegiate playing career, an unanticipated transition might be suffering a season-ending injury, and a non-event might be not receiving necessary coach feedback.

In any case, it is not the transition itself that influences athletes' psychosocial response, but rather their interpretation/appraisal of the transition (Schlossberg, 1981). She noted several dichotomous factors influencing individuals' transition perception, including role change (i.e., gaining vs. losing something), affect (i.e., positive vs. negative), source (i.e., internal vs. external), timing (i.e., on-time vs. early or late), onset (gradual vs. sudden), and duration (permanent, temporary, or uncertain). To put transition perception into a sporting context—two seniors both coming to the end of their playing career may have drastically different responses depending on whether they emphasize losing their identity as a football player versus gaining an identity as a college graduate and young professional (i.e., role change), and whether they feel that they have accomplished all that they could as an athlete, or that the end has come prematurely and are uncertain about their ability to play professionally (i.e., timing, duration).

In addition to individuals' perception of the transition, the model specifies two other factors mediating the effect of transition type on individual adaptation: (a) pre- and post-transition environmental characteristics (e.g., social support), and (b) characteristics of the individual (e.g., demographics, previous experience). When individuals possess the necessary environmental and individual characteristics to handle the demands of the transition, they can integrate the new circumstances into their life (i.e., positive adaptation). However, if the demands of the transition exceed individuals' resources, psychosocial health may suffer. In returning to the example of the athletes coming to the end of their collegiate playing career, the athlete who has taken advantage of institutional programs aimed at helping to prepare him for life post-sport, and who has confidence in his ability to successfully move on from sport, is likely to fare better than the athlete who has counted on being drafted to play professionally, and sees himself primarily as an athlete. Schlossberg's model offers a coherent explanation of the process of general life transitions. Of course, high-level sport is sufficiently unique to warrant its own line of research on the transitions of athletes. The majority of studies have focused on athletes' transition into sport retirement.

The sport retirement transition

Although isolated studies of athlete transition date to the 1950's, as noted by Wylleman, Alfermann, and Lavallee (2004), many of the earliest studies on the psychosocial aspects of sport adopted a social gerontological and thanatological approach to the issue, which proved insufficient for explaining the retirement experiences of relatively young individuals moving on from the unique subculture of sport and into the larger society. Thus, prior to the development of sport-specific models, Schlossberg's (1981) transition model was a popular framework for the study of athlete transition. Studies in the 1980s and 1990s focused on the sport retirement transition, and enlightened researchers and professionals on the challenges of adjustment to retirement for high-level athletes (Sinclair & Orlick, 1993; Werthner & Orlick, 1986). Notably, retirement from sport was not necessarily viewed as distressful by athletes in these early studies. In fact, athletes who had achieved their sport goals and who left sport on their own terms noted a relatively smooth transition out of sport.

Based on theories of transition in general, and studies of sport retirement published at that time, Taylor and Ogilvie (1994) offered a sport-specific model of athlete retirement. The authors adopted a sequential stage-based model to describe the process of and key milestones characterizing athlete retirement. The first stage focuses on the reason for retirement, which in sport may be any one or a combination of age, deselection, injury, or choice. As presented by Schlossberg (1981), individuals' transition perceptions are partially shaped by whether the transition is anticipated (e.g., age/year in school), unanticipated (e.g., injury), or a non-event (e.g., not being re-signed by a team). Because unanticipated transitions are the most difficult to prepare for, they have the highest probability of turning into a crisis for athletes. The second stage of Taylor and Ogilvie's model highlights the factors influencing athletes' retirement adaptation. They propose that successful adaptation is dependent on the extent to which athletes have been afforded the opportunity for holistic personal development through sport, how deeply their sense of self is tied to sport, how much control they perceive having over their decision to retire, and sociodemographic factors such as socioeconomic status and race/ethnicity.

Similar to Schlossberg's focus on environmental factors influencing transition, in stage three Taylor and Ogilvie highlight the importance of resources such as social support, pre-retirement planning, and coping skills for successful adaptation to retirement. The preceding stages feed into stage four, is the quality of athletes' adaptation to retirement. As initially suggested by Coakley (1983), and supported by Greendorfer and Blinde (1985) and Sinclair and Orlick (1993), Taylor and Ogilvie posit that retirement is not necessarily distressful for athletes. Indeed, if the necessary "ingredients" for positive adaptation are present in stages 2 and 3 (e.g., transferable skills, balanced identity, social support), rather than view retirement as threatening, athletes may instead treat it as a celebration of past accomplishments, and an "opening ceremony" for the next phase of life. The fifth stage of the model refers to pre- and post-retirement interventions aimed toward ensuring a satisfying transition for athletes. In the years since Taylor and Ogilvie's model was published, researchers have more thoroughly examined the influence of retirement on athletes' psychosocial health, including the personal and social antecedents that moderate this process.

Steady interest in athletes' retirement experiences from researchers, combined with an overall increased concern for psychosocial health and well-being in athletes, has recently led to several review articles on athlete career transition which nicely synthesize the current state of knowledge. The first of these reviews was conducted by Park, Lavallee, and Tod (2013), and covered 126 studies on athletes' transition out of sport published between 1968 and 2010. Although most studies focused on elite-level athletes, studies of retirement at all competitive levels were included. The authors noted several trends in findings relevant for the psychosocial health consequences of athlete retirement. Notably, a strong athletic identity, involuntary retirement, the perception that sport goals had not been met, lack of autonomy, poor coach relations, lack of pre-retirement sport-life balance, lack of pre-retirement planning, and lack of psychosocial support were all related to poorer quality of adjustment to retirement. The review by Park et al. validated many facets of Taylor and Ogilvie's (1994) model of sport retirement, and highlighted gaps in the literature for researchers to address. Around the same time,

Fuller (2014) conducted a meta-synthesis of nine qualitative studies on inter-collegiate athletes' transition out of sport conducted between 1988 and 2011. Findings largely supported Park et al., but also elucidated some issues that might be of particular concern for collegiate athletes. For example, loss of camaraderie appeared to be a significant issue for this population, as teammates who once served as a source of emotional support were missed, and athletes were forced to discover new support networks. Another important theme across studies was the notion of gradually "branching out" prior to retirement. That is, athletes who began shifting their focus to other realms of life prior to retirement, such as academics, non-sport social relationships, and new competitive outlets experiences a smoother transition out of intercollegiate sport.

Although the reviews by Park et al. (2013) and Fuller (2014) were useful for identifying the factors influencing athletes' adjustment to retirement, an important but taken-for-granted question in reviews of sport retirement transition and the studies within them is exactly what constitutes "quality" psychosocial adaptation or adjustment of athletes to the exit from sport? As previously mentioned, sport scholars have wisely cautioned against assuming the worst about former athletes' retirement experience merely because they may have moved on to less glamorous jobs and daily activities (Coakley, 1983; Greendorfer & Blinde, 1985). That is, "just because ex-athletes become similar to those they resembled when their sport careers began does not necessarily signal trauma, identity crises, or serious adjustment problems" (Coakley, 1983, p. 10). Indeed, whereas some athletes do experience retirement as a crisis, many more adjust quite well (Stambulova & Wylleman, 2014).

Of course, for many of the reasons already noted, some athletes do truly struggle to adjust to life post-sport. From the 1950s through the 1980s researchers relied mainly on retired athletes' subjective reports of adjustment using interviews, unvalidated questionnaires, or a combination of the two (e.g., Werthner & Orlick, 1986; Kirson Weinberg & Arond, 1952). Although these studies yielded valuable information about athletes' retirement experiences, they did little to help distinguish a healthy/normal response to transition from an unhealthy/abnormal response. Fortunately, researchers have begun employing psychometrically sound measures that allow for more precise inferences about retired athletes' psychosocial health. A recent systematic review by Mannes, et al. (2018) included results of 40 studies conducted between 2000 and 2017 measuring indices of retired elite athletes' emotional health (e.g., depression, anxiety, substance abuse). The primary finding, and one of importance in discussing the psychosocial health implications of athlete retirement, is that the overall rate of psychological distress in former high-level athletes at least two years post-retirement is similar to that of the general population.

However, the review revealed that some athletes seem to be at greater risk for distress in retirement. Illustrating the intersection of injury and transition, depression and substance abuse were more common in retired athletes who reported more injuries, concussions, and substance misuse during their careers, and athletes with a current diagnosis of osteoarthritis. Thus, there seems to be a link between the quality of athletes' physical health and their resultant psychosocial health, which has particular implications for athletes in contact sports such as American football and ice hockey, where collision-related pain and injury are more common. As discussed in Chapter 7, athletes who have experienced head trauma may be prone to cognitive health impairments as well as emotional health issues such as depression and anxiety. Further, athletes who sustained high amounts of physical contact during their playing career may try to self-medicate for their pain. The review by Mannes et al. (2018) is an important contribution relative to psychosocial health and retirement, as it can aid professionals in identifying athletes who might be particularly at risk for poor psychosocial health upon the transition out of sport.

One element of Mannes et al.'s (2018) review warranting attention is their choice to include only studies in which athletes were at least two years post-retirement. Because transition in general, and retirement specifically, is a dynamic process, it can be expected that athletes' psychosocial response will change from the time immediately post-retirement to the ensuing months and years. Thus, it is expected that indicators of psychosocial health immediately post-retirement will change. The few longitudinal investigations of retired athletes that have been conducted suggest that as the time since retirement increases, retired athletes' life satisfaction increases and life stress decreases (e.g., Douglas & Carless, 2009; Wippert & Wippert, 2008). In one study, Stephan, Bilard, Ninot, and Delignières (2003) undertook a mixed-methods investigation of subjective well-being (SWB) in 16 elite athletes at four times during their first year post-retirement. As shown by a combination of interviews and scores on the French version of the General Health Questionnaire, athletes reported an initial decrease in SWB in the two months immediately post-retirement, followed by an improvement and stabilization of SWB between five and eight months, and a final improvement in SWB at 11–12 months post-retirement. Of note is that all of the athletes in the study retired voluntarily, which, according to Taylor and Ogilvie's (1994) model, has implications for the ease with which they adjust.

A study with retired gymnasts by Kerr and Dacyshyn (2000) nicely displays the dynamic nature of athletes' psychosocial responses to sport exit. The authors interviewed seven former elite gymnasts between the ages of 16 and 22 who were between six months and five years post-retirement. Because competitive gymnasts retire particularly young, the authors were interested in the unique challenges associated with retirement in these young women. An inductive analysis of the interviews resulted in three major themes illustrating the process of retirement for the former gymnasts. The first phase of the process was *Retirement*, which consisted of quotes detailing athletes' reason for retirement. Five of the seven gymnasts either retired involuntarily (e.g., injury), or because the sport was no longer enjoyable. The other two gymnasts retired of their own volition upon achieving all their goals in the sport. Regardless of why the gymnasts retired, they reported a sense of loss which Kerr and Dacyshyn (2000) termed *Nowhere Land*. The following quote is illustrative of the athletes' emotions during this phase of retirement:

> I'm just kind of floating around. I always find myself coming back to gymnastics. I'm just hoping to get another focus … I'm adjusted but I won't be happy until I actually get into [another activity].
>
> *(Kerr & Dacyshyn, 2000, p. 123)*

Although some of the gymnasts in the study remained in the previous phase at the time of their interview, several had moved on to a phase that the authors named *New Beginnings*, in which they moved on to different activities such as school, and embraced a new and more balanced identity. Perhaps to be expected, five of the seven gymnasts expressed at least some difficulty with retirement in the beginning. However, in support of retirement as a process, three had successfully moved beyond their struggles. Thus, any discussion of athletes' psychosocial response to retirement should necessarily consider the temporal nature of the experience.

Summary

Because high-level athletes necessarily spend years of their life training to achieve their sport goals, retirement can represent a traumatic event. Based on extant theories of life transition, Taylor and Ogilvie (1994) proposed a model of sport retirement for high-level athletes, which emphasizes factors such as the reasons for retirement, breadth of identity, and socioeconomic status as critical in determining the quality of adaptation to retirement. The ensuing years of research and the results of comprehensive review papers largely support the tenets of Taylor and Ogilvie's model, and offer insight into the factors that place athletes at greater risk for psychosocial health difficulties upon retirement. Further, the results of such studies emphasize the dynamic nature of athletes' psychosocial responses to retirement, as most athletes studied report a period of disorientation immediately following retirement, followed by an eventual rebound of their psychosocial health and well-being.

Within-career sport transitions

In the International Society of Sport Psychology's (ISSP) 2009 position stand on career development and transitions of athletes, Stambulova, Alfermann, Statler, and Côte noted a shift in research beginning in the early 2000's from an almost exclusive focus on the end of athletes' career toward an understanding of within-career sport transitions such as advancing from one competitive level to the next, returning from injury, moving to a new country, or even changing sports. A major contribution to researchers' understanding of within-sport transitions was Wylleman and Lavallee's (2003) developmental model of athlete transitions, which offers a holistic view of the interacting and overlapping transitions (e.g., athletic, psychological, academic/vocational) encountered by athletes from initiation to discontinuation of sport. The model has important implications, as rather than view athletes' psychosocial response to sport transitions in a vacuum, researchers and practitioners must also consider the role of simultaneous and interacting non-sport transitions.

The junior-to-senior level transition (JST) is the most often studied within-career sport transition, as researchers seek to understand the process by which athletes adjust to playing at a higher level of competition. Many athletes face significant difficulty in the change from being a "big fish in a small pond" to a "little fish in a big pond," and up to two-thirds fail to successfully cope with the transition (Pehrson, Stambulova, & Olsson, 2017). Stambulova's (2003) career transition model (CTM), which posits that the outcome of sport transition is dependent on the balance between athletes' coping resources and transition demands, has been widely used to understand the JST. According to the CTM, when athletes' possess sufficient internal (knowledge and skills) and external (social support) resources with which to handle their transition, they will experience a successful transition. However, when demands exceed athletes' resources, they may either experience a delayed adaptation to the transition, or, more long-term disruption to psychosocial health such as anxiety, depression, disordered eating, and substance abuse.

Using both the CTM and the developmental model of sport transition as a guide, Stambulova, Franck, and Weibull (2012) examined the JST in Swedish ice hockey players. They found that athletes' resources (i.e., coping strategies, environmental support) predicted significant variance in sport satisfaction. Thus, as suggested by the CTM, athletes' perceived resources are an important factor in athletes' adjustment to the JST. In support of Wylleman and Lavallee's (2003) holistic conceptualization of sport transition, sport satisfaction positively predicted life satisfaction, and perceived adjustment to the senior level negatively predicted life satisfaction. The latter finding is particularly intriguing, as the authors suggest that athletes' struggle to adjust to a new level of competition may pull them away from other aspects of their life, thereby diminishing satisfaction with life in general, even while sport satisfaction remained strong (Stambulova et al., 2012).

Others have employed the CTM and developmental model to study the experience of young adult and adult athletes transitioning into the elite and professional ranks. Bruner, Munroe-Chandler, and Spink (2008) conducted focus groups with eight male ice hockey players during their first season of Major Junior "A" hockey. In addition to the advancement in competitive level faced by all the athletes, seven of the eight were living away from home for the first time. The players noted several on-ice and off-ice issues related to the transition, and athlete quotes revealed the psychosocial impact of these issues. For example, coach feedback was challenging for some of the players to handle:

> [When] they [the coaches] are criticizing you then you feel like they hate me. I suck out there. But they say they are doing it to make you a better player. It [constructive criticism] is hard to see at that time.
>
> *(Bruner et al., 2008, p. 245)*

Despite their difficulties, all of the athletes had a positive view of the transitions, and unanimously reflected a belief that they were maturing as players and as people.

Whereas nearly all studies of within-sport career transition have been conducted with youth athletes, Sanders and Winter (2016) filled a gap in the literature by studying the transition experience of adult triathletes from the amateur to the professional level. Not surprisingly, these athletes' experience was much different than the ice hockey players studied by Bruner et al. (2008). The social health implications of the athletes' choice were clear in their responses to interview questions. For example, they expressed mixed support from family and friends. Whereas many were supportive, some athletes noted disapproval from family and friends who doubted the financial viability of their plan to compete professionally. Others struggled with the decision to prioritize their triathlon training over socializing with non-triathlete friends. Issues of identity were central to the athletes' transition experience, as many questioned whether they had made the right decision to pursue triathlon professionally, and others seemingly embarrassed to identify as a professional athlete. At the same time, similar to the young ice hockey players, all of the adult triathletes discussed a sense of growth and development due to the transition from amateur to professional.

Summary

Although sport retirement is the most often studied transition of high-level athletes, these individuals also experience numerous transitions within their career that can potentially shape their psychosocial health. Both Wylleman and Lavallee's (2003) developmental model and Stambulova's (2003) CTM have proven valuable for understanding within-career sport transitions, and highlight the complex nature of these events. Studies with youth and adult athletes demonstrate how changes in competitive level can have a broad impact on their lives. Notably, if the necessary personal and environmental resources are present, athletes can experience transition as an opportunity for personal growth and development.

Future research directions

From the perspective of sport transition and psychosocial health in high-level athletes, a number of interesting research questions remain unanswered.

First, because the body is central to athletes' sporting lives, it would be interesting to understand the short- and long-term influence of sport retirement on body image and associated body-change behaviors. Stephan and Bilard (2003) reported negative changes in body satisfaction between 1.5 and 5 months post-retirement in former Olympic athletes. However, the researchers employed a between-groups design comparing body satisfaction in current and retired athletes rather than a longitudinal within-group analysis of change from pre to post-retirement. The latter design is necessary to control for potential group differences, and to understand the before-after body-image effect of retirement from life as a high-level athlete to life as a recreational athlete, exerciser, or sedentary individual.

Second, there is an opportunity to better understand the spiritual health outcomes of sport transition. Because transitions can constitute a fundamental shift in athletes' assumptions about the world and their identity as an athlete, it is natural to consider how such changes affect athletes' sense of connection with a higher power. The role of spirituality in life transition is a current topic of interest in the occupational therapy literature (e.g., Maley, Pagana, Velenger, & Humbert, 2016), but spiritual health has been largely neglected in the study of sport transition. The spiritual dimension may be most relevant for unplanned sport retirement due to illness or injury, as such an untimely exit from sport likely prompts athletes to consider spiritual issues such as life meaning and purpose.

Finally, researchers should consider further embracing a eudaimonic perspective on sport transition and psychosocial health in high-level athletes. That is, rather than equating successful adaptation to transition as the absence of psychopathology or the presence of positive emotions (i.e., subjective well-being), investigators might consider outcomes such as personal growth, life purpose, and self-acceptance (i.e., psychological well-being; Ryff, 1989). It may be that transitioning athletes experience concurrent decrements in subjective well-being and enhancement of psychological well-being. Indeed, the results of qualitative studies suggest that despite the challenges of transition, many athletes do perceive personal growth and development consistent with psychological well-being (e.g., Bruner et al., 2008; Sanders & Winter, 2016).

Conclusion

Depending on environmental context and personal resources, transition has the potential to prompt psychosocial health enhancement or debilitation. Social gerontological and thanatological approaches, as well as general psychosocial models of life transition, have been abandoned in favor of sport-specific frameworks outlining the necessary conditions for successful adaptation to transition for athletes (e.g., Stambulova, 2003; Taylor & Ogilvie, 1994; Wylleman & Lavallee, 2003). Although the prevalence of psychological distress is similar between retired athletes and the general population, athletes who experienced high amounts of pain, injury, and blows to the head during their career may be more susceptible to emotional health concerns. Further research is necessary to understand specific psychosocial facets of athletes' transition experience, as well as the interplay of hedonic and eudaimonic indicators of well-being.

References

Bruner, M. W., Munroe-Chandler, K. J., & Spink, K. S. (2008). Entry into elite sport: A preliminary investigation into the transition experiences of rookie athletes. *Journal of Applied Sport Psychology, 20*(2), 236–252. doi:10.1080/10413200701867745

Coakley, J. J. (1983). Leaving competitive sport: Retirement or rebirth? *Quest, 35*(1), 1–11. doi:10.1080/00336297.1983.10483777

Douglas, K., & Carless, D. (2009). Abandoning the performance narrative: Two women's stories of transition from professional sport. *Journal of Applied Sport Psychology, 21*(2), 213–230. doi:10.1080/10413200902795109

Franck, A., & Stambulova, N. (2017). A Swedish female basketball player's junior-to-senior transition: A narrative case study. In K. Hertting & U. Johnson (Eds.), *Proceedings of the Nordic Sport Science Conference—The double-edged sword of sport: Health promotion versus unhealthy environments* (pp. 32–33). Halmstad, Sweden: Halmstad University Press.

Fuller, R. D. (2014). Transition experiences out of intercollegiate athletics: A metasynthesis. *The Qualitative Report, 19*(46), 1–15. Retrieved from https://nsuworks. nova.edu/tqr/vol19/iss46/1

Greendorfer, S. L., & Blinde, E. M. (1985). "Retirement" from intercollegiate sport: Theoretical and empirical considerations. *Sociology of Sport Journal, 2*(2), 101–110. doi:10.1123/ssj.2.2.101

Janoff-Bulman, R. (2002). Shattered assumptions: Towards a new psychology of trauma. New York, NY: Free Press.

Kerr, G., & Dacyshyn, A. (2000). The retirement experiences of elite, female gymnasts. *Journal of Applied Sport Psychology, 12*(2), 115–133. doi:10.1080/10413200008404218

Kirson Weinberg, S. & Arond, H. (1952). The occupational culture of the boxer. *American Journal of Sociology, 57*, 460–469. Retrieved from https://www.jstor.org/ stable/2772326

Liekas, S., & Salmela-Aro, K. (2014). Personality types during transition to young adulthood: How are they related to life situation and well-being? *Journal of Adolescence, 37*, 753–762. doi:10.1016/j.adolescence.2014.01.003

Maley, C. M., Pagana, N. K., Velenger, C. A., & Humbert, T. K. (2016). Dealing with major life events and transitions: A systematic literature review on and occupational analysis of spirituality. *American Journal of Occupational Therapy, 70*(4). doi:10.5014/ ajot.2016.015537

Mannes, Z. L., Waxenberg, L. B., Cottler, L. B., Perlstein, W. M., Burrell, L. E., II, Ferguson, E. G., … Ennis, N. (2018). Prevalence and correlates of psychological distress among retired elite athletes: A systematic review. *International Review of Sport and Exercise Psychology.* doi:10.1080/1750984X.2018.1469162

Park, S., Lavallee, D., & Tod, D. (2013). Athletes' career transition out of sport: A systematic review. *International Review of Sport and Exercise Psychology, 6*(1), 22–53. doi:10.1080/1750984X.2012.687053

Parkes, C. M. (1971). Psycho-social transitions: A field for study. *Social Science & Medicine, 5*(2), 101–115. doi:10.1016/0037-7856(71)90091-6

Pehrson, S., Stambulova, N. B., & Olsson, K. (2017). Revisiting the empirical model "Phases in the junior-to-senior transition of Swedish ice hockey players": External validation through focus groups and interviews. *International Journal of Sports Science & Coaching, 12*(6), 747–761. doi:10.1177/1747954117738897

Sanders, P., & Winter, S. (2016). Going pro: Exploring adult triathletes' transitions into elite sport. *Sport, Exercise, and Performance Psychology, 5*(3), 193–205. doi:10.1037/spy0000058

Schlossberg, N. K. (1981). A model for analyzing human adaptation to transition. *The Counseling Psychologist, 9*(2), 2–18. doi:10.1177/001100008100900202

Sinclair, D., & Orlick, T. (1993). Positive transitions from high-performance sport. *The Sport Psychologist, 7,* 138–150. doi:10.1123/tsp.7.2.138

Stambulova, N. (2003). Symptoms of a crisis-transition: A grounded theory study. In *Årsbok: Svensk idrottspsykologisk förening [Yearbook: Swedish Sports Psychological Association]* (pp. 97–109). Örebro, Sweden: Svensk idrottspsykologisk förening [Swedish Sports Psychological Association].

Stambulova, N. B. (2017). Crisis-transitions in athletes: Current emphases on cognitive and contextual factors. *Current Opinion in Psychology, 16,* 62–66. doi:10.1016/j.copsyc.2017.04.013

Stambulova, N., Alfermann, D., Statler, T., & Côté, J. (2009). ISSP position stand: Career development and transitions of athletes. *International Journal of Sport and Exercise Psychology, 7*(4), 395–412. doi:10.1080/1612197X.2009.9671916

Stambulova, N., Franck, A., & Weibull, F. (2012). Assessment of the transition from junior-to-senior sports in Swedish athletes. *International Journal of Sport and Exercise Psychology, 10*(2), 79–95. doi:10.1080/1612197X.2012.645136

Stambulova, N., & Wylleman, P. (2014). Athletes' career development and transitions. In A. G. Papaioannou & D. Hackfort (Eds.), *International perspectives on key issues in sport and exercise psychology. Routledge companion to sport and exercise psychology: Global perspectives and fundamental concepts* (pp. 605–620). New York, NY: Routledge/Taylor & Francis Group.

Stephan, Y., & Bilard, J. (2003). Repercussions of transition out of elite sport on body image. *Perceptual and Motor Skills, 96*(1), 95–104. doi:10.2466/pms.2003.96.1.95

Stephan, Y., Bilard, J., Ninot, G., & Delignières, D. (2003). Bodily transition out of elite sport: A one-year study of physical self and global self-esteem among transitional athletes. *International Journal of Sport and Exercise Psychology, 1*(2), 192–207. doi:10.1080/1612197X.2003.9671712

Taylor, J., & Ogilvie, B. C. (1994). A conceptual model of adaptation to retirement among athletes. *Journal of Applied Sport Psychology, 6*(1), 1–20. doi:10.1080/10413209408406462

transition. (2018). In *Merriam Webster.* Retrieved from https://www.merriam-webster.com/dictionary/transition

Werthner, P., & Orlick, T. (1986). Retirement experiences of successful Olympic athletes. *International Journal of Sport Psychology, 17*(5), 337–363.

Wippert, P.-M., & Wippert, J. (2008). Perceived stress and prevalence of traumatic stress symptoms following athletic career termination. *Journal of Clinical Sport Psychology, 2*(1), 1–16. doi:10.1123/jcsp.2.1.1

Wylleman, P., Alfermann, D., & Lavallee, D. (2004). Career transitions in sport: European perspectives. *Psychology of Sport and Exercise, 5*(1), 7–20. doi:10.1016/S1469-0292(02)00049-3

Wylleman, P., & Lavallee, D. (2003). A developmental perspective on transitions faced by athletes. In M. Weiss (Ed.), *Developmental sport and exercise psychology: A lifespan perspective* (pp. 507–527). Morgantown, WV: Fitness Information Technology.

PART III

Interventions and positive outcomes

Although threats to athletes' psychosocial health are inevitable, their effects can be prevented and managed. Many athletes seem to quickly bounce back from adversity, and some even emerge better than they were before. In this final part I address the prevention and treatment of psychosocial health concerns in high-level athletes, as well as the potential for resilience and growth due to threats in the sport environment. In *Chapter 9*, I draw heavily from research in the field of public health to make a case for the power of prevention. In addition to orienting readers to the fundamental aspects of prevention, I review and critique programs that have been implemented by high-level sport organizations. I continue making parallels with public health in *Chapter 10* when I discuss how policy can be used to forward comprehensive prevention efforts in sport. As part of the policy discussion, I highlight and comment on a few of the policies already in place for enhancing athletes' psychosocial health.

In *Chapter 11*, I focus on common approaches to the treatment of psychosocial health issues in athletes, including psychotherapeutic interventions and support groups. I note the unique challenges that accompany treatment in high-level athletes, as well as the lack of rigorous and large-scale evaluation of treatment efforts. I close the section in *Chapter 12* with a discussion of the conditions under which athletes successfully adapt to threats in the sport environment, or in some cases experience growth *because* of them. After a brief historical overview of research on resilience and adversarial growth in non-athletes, I highlight recent advances in the study of these constructs in high-level athletes, and conclude with evidence-based recommendations for empowering athletes with the tools and environments necessary for resilience and growth to occur.

9

PREVENTION

Concerned by several recent incidents of off-field misbehavior, and an uptick in players requesting mental health services due to on- and off-field stressors, Sharon, who is the director of athlete development for a professional sport club, has decided that rather than devote most of her resources toward after-the-fact services for struggling athletes, it would be wise to take a more pro-active approach by also investing in initiatives focused on early risk-detection and athlete empowerment. Upon a thorough needs assessment in which she gathered quantitative data, observed day-to-day activities, and interviewed players and staff, Sharon determines that a two-tiered prevention approach is the best fit for her club. The first tier will involve mandatory life-skills training (e.g., stress management, social responsibility, financial management) for *all* first-year players over the course of their entire rookie season. As part of this tier, every first-year player will be paired with a veteran on the team who can support them in making a successful transition to professional sport. Sharon hopes that the successful implementation of tier-one prevention will drastically reduce instances of later athlete trouble and distress. Sharon recognizes that certain athletes may require more extensive or specialized services, which is why she will institute a second tier to her plan, designed to target athletes that research suggests are at higher than average risk to struggle with the transition to professional sport. One group of special interest is foreign-born players, who must not only adapt to their new career, but a new country and language as well. In addition to the tier-one services offered to all players, foreign-born players will have the option to receive tier-two services to aid in their adjustment to life in their new country.

Throughout Part II I detailed some of the more common threats to high-level athletes' psychosocial health. Recent high-profile cases of psychosocial health concerns in athletes have prompted sport-governing bodies to initiate programming aimed at addressing threats and preventing psychosocial ill-being. In this chapter I highlight several programs designed either to prevent the occurrence of threats to athletes' psychosocial health and/or mitigate the effect of these threats on psychosocial health.

The language and logic of prevention

Before discussing specific prevention programs for athletes, it is first necessary to define the term, as well as others closely associated with it. Most simply, *prevention* references efforts made to ensure that something does not happen. Much of what professionals know about prevention is credited to the work of researchers interested in the factors associated with substance abuse and child psychopathology (e.g., Garmezy, 1993; Hawkins, Catalano, & Miller, 1992). In the context of addiction, mental illness, and other public health issues, Bloom (1996) offered the following definition of prevention:

> Coordinated actions seeking to prevent predictable problems, to protect existing states of health and healthy functioning and to promote desired potentialities in individuals and groups in their physical and sociocultural settings over time.
>
> *(p. 2)*

Most prevention efforts are aimed at either reducing *risk factors* and *vulnerability factors*, or enhancing *protective factors* and *resilience factors* (Begun, 1993). Risk and protective factors are those present in the social and environmental that either increase (i.e., risk) or decrease (i.e., protective) the probability of adverse health outcomes. Within high-level youth sport, a hostile and abusive coach might be a risk factor for anxiety and depression in young athletes. By contrast, a protective factor for adverse emotional health might be the presence of a variety of on-campus resources for athletes such as academic advising and the counseling center. By contrast, vulnerability and resilience factors are attributes intrinsic to individuals (e.g., biology, personality) that either heighten (i.e., vulnerability) or dampen (i.e., resilience) the likelihood of health concerns. Whereas an athlete with a family history of addiction might be more vulnerable to substance abuse, an athlete with a strong internal locus of control might be resilient to stressful conditions that might otherwise lead to substance abuse. Of course, people don't exist in a vacuum, and psychosocial health is ultimately determined by a complex interplay of all four factors.

Historically studied and employed in the context of averting physical disease, the benefits of before-the-fact prevention versus after-the-fact treatment have been hotly debated (Woolf, Husten, Lewin, Marks, Fielding, & Sanchez, 2009).

In addition to the enhanced quality of life that arises from not having to experience or treat a given health concern, proponents of preventive healthcare frequently cite economic benefits as a primary benefit of prevention. For example, Levi, Segal, and Juliano (2008) reported a potential return on investment of 5.60:1 if $10 per person per year was spent on evidence-based prevention programs focused on physical activity, smoking, nutritional practices, and participation in routine health screenings. As alluded to in the Trust for America report, the concept of prevention has expanded in recent years to include practices used at various stages of disease progression, as well as those aimed at overall well-being and risky health behaviors (Starfield, Hyde, Gérvas, & Heath, 2008). A contemporary perspective on prevention comes from The American College of Preventive Medicine (ACPM), which states that the goal of preventive medicine is to "protect, promote, and maintain health and well-being and to prevent disease, disability, and death" (ACPM, n.d., para. 1). The ACPM statement illustrates how conceptualizations of prevention have broadened to include the promotion and maintenance of health in addition to disease prevention. Further, Woolf et al. (2009) noted how notions of prevention have evolved from a focus on preventing diseases themselves (e.g., Diabetes) to preventing behaviors strongly associated with disease (e.g., physical inactivity).

Two classifications have been widely adopted by researchers and practitioners when discussing prevention. The first and most common taxonomy was offered by Morris (1957) and classifies prevention practices based on the period of time in which they are implemented. Using the Commission's taxonomy, prevention can be *primary* (i.e., acting to prevent a problem before it occurs), *secondary* (i.e., acting in the early stages of a problem to prevent it from worsening), or *tertiary* (i.e., managing a chronic problem and/or minimizing negative consequences). To contextualize the three types of prevention in the sport realm, primary prevention of concussion in American football might include investing in quality safety equipment such as helmets and pads, as well as teaching proper tackling mechanics. Secondary prevention would occur following a blow to the head, and would include the assessment of players' cognitive function, coordination, and balance on the sideline by trained medical staff. Tertiary prevention refers to ongoing symptom management and return to activity as appropriate.

Although the primary-secondary-tertiary taxonomy is widely used, some have noted inconsistencies in usage and overlap between the three categories. In response to the weaknesses of the Commission's taxonomy, Gordon (1987) proposed a framework of prevention based on characteristics of the population served. Within Gordon's framework, *universal* prevention refers to initiatives aimed at the entire population, and for which the potential benefits of the prevention practice outweigh the cost of participating in the initiative. *Selective* prevention is used for individuals who have a higher than average risk of developing a health problem. Finally, *indicated* prevention is employed when individuals are at high risk for a health problem. Within sport, a universal prevention initiative might occur when all rookie athletes in a professional league receive education and support for the transition into professional sport. Selective prevention might be a special seminar or group for teenage athletes making the transition. Finally, once the season begins, an indicated prevention approach such as one-on-one counseling might be necessary for athletes exhibiting signs of poor psychosocial adjustment to the transition.

A more holistic framework for prevention was proposed by Weisz, Sandler, Durlak, and Anton (2005), who applied Gordon's (1987) taxonomy to interventions employed both prior to and following the presence of symptomatology. In addition to the original universal-selective-indicated intervention categories, Weisz et al. suggested categories for *health promotion/positive development* strategies and *treatment interventions*. The former refers to population-wide efforts to foster personal strengths rather than reduce risk factors, and the latter refers to intervention for individuals who exhibit advanced symptoms and/or have been formally diagnosed with a clinical disorder. A strengths-based approach to prevention aligns with the positive psychology and positive health movements which gained popularity in the early 2000s and have been influential in the development of various prevention programs since this time. In the remainder of this chapter I highlight and critique initiatives focused on bolstering strengths, as well as those adopting a universal and selective prevention approach. Indicated prevention and treatment are discussed in Chapter 10.

Health promotion/positive development and universal prevention for athletes

As previously discussed, both universal prevention and health promotion/positive development approaches are designed to positively influence entire populations rather than specific sub-groups of individuals. Thus, for this section, I focus on interventions, programs, and strategies aimed at high-level athletes in general. The difference between universal and health promotion/positive development lies in the intervention goal. Whereas universal prevention efforts are designed to reduce unwanted risk and vulnerability factors, health promotion/positive development strategies are designed to leverage and enhance desirable protective and resilience factors leading to positive outcomes. The latter approach has long been promoted as important by sport psychology professionals who argue that the goals of high-level sport should extend beyond performance success to include personal development (e.g., Danish, Petitpas, & Hale, 1992; Miller & Kerr, 2002). There have been two major targets for psychosocial-focused health promotion and universal prevention interventions and strategies in high-level athletes: (a) substance abuse and (b) stress.

Because college athletes report higher rates of alcohol use than their non-athlete peers, (Wechsler, Davenport, Dowdall, Grossman, & Zanakos, 1997), researchers have taken an interest in developing, implementing, and evaluating interventions aimed at reducing athlete drinking. Noting that college athletes tend to overestimate the extent to which peers drink alcohol, thereby leading to efforts to mimic the perceived drinking behavior of these same peers, Thombs and Hamilton (2002) undertook a universal prevention program aimed at altering collegiate athletes' perceptions of their peers' drinking behavior. The researchers launched a social norm feedback campaign, including bus signage, ads in the campus newspaper, table tents, classroom presentations, and mass mailings designed to correct student-athletes' perceptions of peer drinking behavior. Although the campaign was successful in altering many of the student-athletes' perceptions (e.g., drinking by teammates, team captains, typical students in general), perceptions of drinking by student-athletes' closest friends were not affected by the campaign. More importantly, student-athletes exposed to the campaign did not drink significantly less than non-exposed student-athletes at other universities. The authors suggested that future social norm interventions target more personal and perhaps non-sport social groups as a way of reducing student-athlete drinking.

As the internet has become more central in shaping college students' and student-athletes' health attitudes and behaviors, researchers have shifted their prevention efforts to web-based platforms (e.g., Doumas, Haustveit, & Coll, 2010; Martens, Kilmer, Beck, & Zamboanga, 2010). More recently, Fearnow-Kenney et al. (2016) implemented and evaluated a web-based alcohol prevention program (i.e., myPlaybook) focused on altering student-athletes' perceptions of social norms, their expectations (positive or negative) about the consequences of drinking, and intention to drink less and/or limit potential harm associated with drinking. As compared to a delayed treatment control group, the student-athletes who received myPlaybook reported more conservative beliefs about peers' drinking, and no decrease in intention to reduce harm related to drinking. Thus, although myPlaybook did not demonstrate changes in actual drinking behavior in student-athletes, it did show positive changes in variables previously shown to mediate the effect of prevention programming on eventual behavior.

Although long discussed (e.g., Buceta, 1985; Smith, 1986), it was not until recently that investigators sought to develop and evaluate universal prevention interventions to reduce negative effects of stress, and relatedly, burnout in high-level athletes. Often termed stress *management*, the goal of most stress-focused interventions is not necessarily to eliminate stress, but rather to teach athletes strategies for effectively handling stressors. Thus, most stress management interventions are best described as adopting a health promotion/positive development approach. In a helpful synthesis of athlete-focused stress management interventions conducted between 1980 and 2010, Rumbold, Fletcher, and Daniels (2012) noted positive effects in 81% of studies primarily focused on stress reduction. A recent contribution to the athlete stress-focused universal prevention literature is a study by Dallmann, Bach, Zipser, Thomann, and Herpertz (2016), in which the authors developed and implemented a six-session stress prevention program with 28 elite adolescent German athletes from a variety of sports. Program content and methods were drawn from the extant literature on stress management, sport-specific risk factors for burnout, and interviews with key sport personnel (e.g., sport psychologists, coaches). Athletes were taught various cognitive and somatic strategies for managing stress (e.g., muscle relaxation, imagery). The program also included mindfulness-based strategies and a discussion of motivation. As compared to the no-intervention control group, the athletes who received the intervention reported a significant increase in stress-related knowledge. However, the stress prevention intervention did not have a significant influence on self-efficacy perceptions of stress. The authors acknowledged several limitations with their intervention, including non-randomization of participants, and a relatively small sample. They suggested further evaluation of their program using a stronger research design.

Although some researchers are interested in stress as an outcome, because poorly managed stress is linked to a variety of deleterious outcomes, others have examined the effect of stress management interventions on undesirable consequences such as sport injury and burnout. Perna, Antoni, Baum, Gordon, and Schneiderman (2003), investigated the effect of a three-week, seven-session cognitive behavioral stress management program on the frequency of injury and illness in a single team of collegiate rowers. The intervention was heavily based on a stress-inoculation training framework, as athletes were trained on a variety of somatic (e.g., progressive muscle relaxation) and cognitive (e.g., imagery) strategies for managing stressful situations in the sport environment. As hypothesized, the athletes randomly assigned to the stress management program experienced significantly fewer days missed due to injury and illness than the control group, who received a single two-hour educational session on stress management. Perna et al.'s findings support the basic tenets of Andersen and Williams' (1988) model of stress and sport injury, as athletes who are equipped to manage stressors may be less likely to become distracted during competition, as well as engage in lifestyle behaviors conducive to injury prevention.

Mindfulness-based approaches to injury prevention, with their emphasis on present-moment and non-judgmental awareness, are an alternative approach to addressing both the stress and attentional components of Andersen and Williams' (1988) stress-injury model. Ivarsson, Johnson, Andersen, Fallby, and Altemyr (2015) tested the efficacy of seven-session mindfulness, acceptance, and commitment (MAC; Gardner & Moore, 2007) program for injury prevention in elite junior Swedish soccer players. Whereas players in a matched control group received seven sessions focused on general sport psychology topics (e.g., team cohesion, motivation), players in the MAC group were educated on mindfulness, acceptance, and commitment, and taught how to apply these concepts in their life. Although group comparison analysis failed to show significant differences, the players in the MAC group experienced fewer total injuries and days lost due to injury than those in the control group. Despite the limitations of the study (e.g., low statistical power, possible cross-contamination, lack of fidelity check), mindfulness-based interventions represent a promising psychological approach to stress management and injury prevention.

Although formal and systematic stress prevention programming is important for optimal psychosocial health in high-level athletes, such programs may be enhanced by the integration of prevention strategies within athletes' day-to-day training. As such, Kroshus and DeFreese (2017) surveyed 933 head collegiate women's soccer coaches regarding their personal efforts to prevent athlete burn-out. Of the coaches who indicated that they intentionally took action to prevent burnout in their athletes, the most commonly employed strategy was limiting physical stressors (e.g., extra days off). Other coaches reported non-physically focused strategies, such as making practice fun, and helping athletes maintain a balanced perspective on sport. Researchers would be wise to consider these more "grass roots" preventive efforts in conjunction with more didactic approaches to stress management/prevention in high-level athletes.

Selective prevention for athletes

In addition to the psychosocial health threats encountered by high-level athletes universally, some threats are gender-specific, unique to athletes in certain sports, or at certain periods of time in their career. As discussed earlier, selective prevention involves identifying a subset of a given population deemed at higher than average risk for one or more health issues. Because of the weight and body-shape demands of certain sports, and gender-specific weight and body pressures, several researchers have developed programs to enhance body satisfaction and/or reduce disordered eating and body-change behaviors. Two programs, Athletes Training and Learning to Avoid Steroids (ATLAS), and Athletes Targeting Healthy Exercise and Nutrition Alternatives (ATHENA), are designed to promote positive body image and healthy weight-management behaviors in adolescent male and female athletes, respectively (Goldberg & Elliot, 2005). Whereas ATLAS targets anabolic steroid abuse, the use of muscle-building supplements, and critiques the "win-at-all-costs" mindset, ATHENA emphasizes self-esteem, prevention of depression, and critiques societal messages around being thin (Goldberg & Elliot, 2005). The defining features of both programs are: (a) the team setting, (b) single-gender delivery, (c) use of peer teachers, and (d) coach facilitation. Both ATLAS and ATHENA are delivered across eight to ten 45-minute coach- and team-leader-led sessions, and feature role play, interactive games, student-created campaigns, and self-monitoring of nutrition as strategies to promote healthy body-related attitudes and behaviors (Goldberg & Elliot, 2005).

Randomized pre-post trials with both the ATLAS and ATHENA programs have yielded promising results. Across two studies, male football players who received the ATLAS intervention reported more knowledge about steroids, improved drug-refusal skills, better nutrition and exercise behaviors, less intention to use steroids, less drinking and driving, and less use of illicit drugs and sport supplements compared to a matched control group (Goldberg, et al., 1996; Goldberg, MacKinnon, Elliot, Moe, Clark, & Cheong, 2000). The ATHENA program has yielded similarly positive results, as female athletes exposed to the program report less use of diet pills and sport supplements, and less intention to use tobacco, vomit for weight loss, or use muscle-building supplements compared to matched controls (Elliot et al., 2008). Intentions to engage in positive health behaviors resulting from ATHENA are mediated both by athletes' perceptions of social norms around ideal body weight and shape, and self-efficacy for eating to become a better athlete (Ranby, et al., 2009). Perhaps most impressively, compared to individuals who did not participate in ATHENA, those who did reported significantly less use of cigarettes, alcohol, and marijuana from one to three years post-graduation. As compared to most sport-based prevention programs, ATLAS and ATHENA programs are unique in that they are grounded in research and theory and have been subjected to rigorous randomized controlled trials with multiple large samples of athletes. Other selective interventions focused on body image and disordered eating have a much smaller base of evidence (Bar, Cassin, & Dionne, 2016).

In their recent review of eating disorder prevention initiatives for athletes, Bar et al. (2016) noted 11 different prevention programs focused on prevention of eating disorders and associated factors (e.g., body satisfaction, negative affect) between 1995 and 2014. The majority of the interventions targeted female athletes in high-risk sports such as dance, gymnastics, and cheerleading. Although positive effects on eating behaviors and body image were found for most interventions, Bar et al. noted several features of the most effective programs: (a) inclusion of coaches and sport administrators in addition to athletes, and (b) interaction across multiple modes of communication, such as peer-led sessions, and use of web-based tools such as social media.

Regarding the latter, Voelker and Petrie's (2017) *Bodies in Motion* program made use of social media as a supplement to regular 75-minute classroom sessions focused on promoting cognitive dissonance and self-compassion as a means of enhancing body image in collegiate female athletes. Athletes were instructed to use social media to not only disseminate messages of body acceptance, but critique online portrayals of women and female athletes' bodies (Voelker & Petrie, 2017). Overall, the program was successful, as athletes who received the intervention reported more positive body image (e.g., body appreciation, body shape concerns) and higher subjective well-being (e.g., happiness, pride) compared to athletes in the control group. Further, many of these differences were sustained three to four months post-intervention. Although it awaits testing with larger samples and across longer periods of time, *Bodies in Motion* fills a gap in being one of the few evidence-based healthy body image promotion/eating disorder prevention programs for college athletes.

Sport organization-developed prevention programming for athletes

In addition to the work of independent researchers, numerous high-level sport governing bodies and organizations have developed and implemented their own programs to prevent psychosocial health concerns and promote well-being in athletes. Although most such programs have not been subject to scientific scrutiny, because of their widespread adoption by high-level sport organizations, I highlight some of them here.

Because of the wide-ranging and intense demands associated with being a student-athlete, combined with a mission of overall personal development, collegiate sport organizations are at the forefront of universal prevention and positive development for athletes. The National Collegiate Athletic Association (NCAA) Life Skills (formerly CHAMPS Life Skills), is the cornerstone athlete development program for the NCAA, which is the largest governing body for collegiate sport in the world. Based on a program created by Dr. Homer Rice, former Athletics Director at Georgia Tech University, NCAA Life Skills, is grounded in the belief that excellent athletes are those who thrive not only athletically, but also academically and personally (NCAA, n.d.). Although member institutions have some degree of autonomy regarding program implementation, all are guided by the NCAA's core commitments to academic excellence, athletic excellence, personal development, career development, and service. For example, the State University of New York Polytechnic University (SUNY Poly) works to fulfill the five commitments through a program called C.A.T.S. (Challenging Athletes to Succeed; SUNY Polytechnic Institute Athletics, n.d.). C.A.T.S. addressed each of the five commitments through a combination of tutoring, workshops, on-campus resources (e.g., dining hall, fitness center, and wellness center), and opportunities for community engagement. Despite widespread adoption of NCAA Life Skills at university athletics departments throughout the U.S., other than a doctoral project by Goddard (2004) showing positive perceptions of the program by student-athletes, there are no published studies of the effectiveness of NCAA Life Skills in any of the five areas of commitment.

Spurred by reports of sexual misconduct at the hands of coaches and other sport personnel, the USOC formed the U.S. Center for SafeSport to prevent and eliminate bullying, hazing, and all forms of abuse in sport (Who We Are, 2018). In addition to serving as the official reporting entity for instances of abuse in all USOC sanctioned sports, SafeSport also offers a web-based training program for all USOC athletes, coaches, and staff. The online modules educate individuals on recognizing and reporting sexual, emotional, and physical misconduct within the sport setting. Module users read about or watch videos related to abuse in sport, as well as vignettes illustrating concepts in practice. At the end of each module, users must pass a test related to the material to receive a SafeSport certificate. Although it is promising that all athletes and personnel are being exposed to content related to abuse, to the extent that the SafeSport training emphasizes knowledge enhancement rather than higher-order learning (e.g., skill-building, opportunities for practice), it is likely to fall short of expectations (Centers for Disease Control and Prevention, 2015).

Selective prevention programs sponsored by sport organizations often focus on the transition into a higher level of sport for young athletes. For example, the

National Basketball Association's (NBA) Rookie Transition Program is a four-day workshop designed to assist rookies in making informed choices related to relevant issues such as sexual relationships, finances, retirement planning, and nutrition (Krawczynski, 2015). Players in the program participate in large and small group settings and learn from a combination of league officials, outside professionals, and former players. Following the admission of emotional health struggles from players such as Kevin Love, a more recent addition to the program is a focus on mental and emotional wellness. As part of the NBA's mental wellness initiative, the league began collaborating with the meditation app Headspace in 2018 to offer complimentary and basketball-specific content to all NBA players and employees (Aldridge, 2018; MacMullan, 2018). Similar to the NBA, in 2016 the National Football League (NFL) began offering a Rookie Transition Program for all drafted and undrafted first-year players. Rather than occurring at a league-wide level, each NFL club is responsible for delivering the three-day orientation. As opposed to the NBA, much of the required content present in the NFL's transition program focuses on logistical (e.g., player benefits, media responsibilities) and on-field issues (e.g., rule changes from college football to the NFL). However, each team must include a focus on social responsibility (e.g., domestic violence, driving under the influence) and mental health.

Future directions

Despite growing interest in the psychosocial health and well-being of high-level athletes, there is a decided lack of well-tested programs for health promotion and early-stage prevention. The few programs that have shown promise in terms of stress reduction or substance abuse prevention have yet to be evaluated on a large scale. The programs that have been widely adopted by large high-level sport organizations such as the NCAA lack theoretical grounding and empirical support. Given the cost of time and money associated with the development and widespread implementation of health promotion and problem prevention programs, it seems imperative that such programs be subject to scientific scrutiny. Within the field of public health promotion, program evaluation is viewed as critical for understanding whether a given program was implemented as intended, if goals were achieved and can be directly attributed to the program, and the efficiency and cost-effectiveness of the program (U.S. Department of Health and Human Services, Centers for Disease Control and Prevention, & Office of the Director, Office of Strategy and Innovation, 2011).

Despite their limitations for evaluating public health programs (e.g., Tones, 2000), the randomized controlled trial (RCT) remains the strongest method for program evaluation, and sport administrators would be wise to subject their program to such an approach. In defending the use of RCTs for health promotion programs, Rosen, Manor, Engelhard, and Zucker (2006) recommend several strategies for conducting RCTs with health promotion programs, including measuring simple outcomes, considering changes in attitudes and beliefs as viable outcomes, randomizing groups (or clusters) rather than individuals, and testing flexible interventions. For example, in conducting an RCT for the NCAA Life Skills program, researchers may choose to measure changes in athletes' attitudes toward community service from before to after the program as compared to a matched group of athletes receiving an alternative program. Further, athletes could be randomized in clusters (e.g., universities) rather than at the individual level to control for possible cross-contamination that may occur if individuals at the same institution were assigned to different groups. Finally, because needs, challenges, and resources of vary, rather than test the exact same program across universities, active participation by student-athletes in the design and implementation of the Life Skills program at their institution can be built into the process of the intervention. Of course, for individual researchers, significant financial resources are necessary to carry out high-quality research. Grant programs such as the NCAA's Innovation in Research and Practice, which awards $100,000 annually to fund applied research projects aimed at student-athlete well-being, will be critical for the continued development of health promotion, universal prevention, and selective prevention programs for high-level athletes.

Conclusion

As awareness of the various threats to psychosocial health in high-level athletes grows, researchers and sport administrators are increasingly interested in early-stage interventions designed to promote positive development and/or prevent deleterious psychosocial health outcomes in athletes. Although some independent researchers have developed and tested universal and selective prevention programs for athletes, except for the ATLAS and ATHENA programs, none have been tested on a large scale. Lack of thorough program evaluation has not precluded several notable sport organizations in the U.S., such as the NCAA, USOC, NBA, and NFL, from requiring athletes and staff to participate in their own "in-house" prevention programs. Although on the surface such programs appear useful, given the time and money spent on development and implementation, data to support (or refute) their effectiveness is warranted. Funding from sources such as the NCAA is critical to support the planning, implementation, and evaluation of high-quality health promotion and problem prevention programs for high-level athletes.

References

Aldridge, D. (2018). *NBA, NBPA taking steps to further address mental wellness issues for players: Independently run mental-wellness program will be funded by league, union.* Retrieved from http://www.nba.com/article/2018/03/12/morning-tip-nba-nbpa-addressing-mental-wellness-issues

American College of Preventive Medicine. (n.d.). *Preventive medicine.* Retrieved from https://www.acpm.org/page/preventivemedicine

Andersen, M. B., & Williams, J. M. (1988). A model of stress and athletic injury: Prediction and prevention. *Journal of Sport and Exercise Psychology, 10*(3), 294–306. doi:10.1123/jsep.10.3.294

Bar, R. J., Cassin, S. E., & Dionne, M. M. (2016). Eating disorder prevention initiatives for athletes: A review. *European Journal of Sport Science, 16*(3), 325–335. doi:10.1080/17461391.2015.1013995

Begun, A. L. (1993). Human behavior and the social environment. *Journal of Social Work Education, 29*(1), 26–35. doi:10.1080/10437797.1993.10778796

Bloom, M. (1996). *Primary prevention practices: Issues in children's and families' lives* (Vol. 5). Thousand Oaks, CA. SAGE.

Buceta, J. M. (1985). Some guidelines for the prevention of excessive stress in athletes. *International Journal of Sport Psychology, 16*(1), 46–58.

Centers for Disease Control and Prevention. (2015). *Characteristics of an effective health education curriculum.* Retrieved from https://www.cdc.gov/healthyschools/sher/characteristics/index.htm

Dallmann, P., Bach, C., Zipser, H., Thomann, P. A., & Herpertz, S. C. (2016). Evaluation of a stress prevention program for young high-performance athletes. *Mental Health & Prevention, 4*(2), 75–80. doi:10.1016/j.mhp.2016.04.001

Danish, S. J., Petitpas, A. J., & Hale, B. D. (1992). A developmental–educational intervention model of sport psychology. *The Sport Psychologist, 6*(4), 403–415. doi:10.1123/tsp.6.4.403

Doumas, D. M., Haustveit, T., & Coll, K. M. (2010). Reducing heavy drinking among first year intercollegiate athletes: A randomized controlled trial of Web-based normative feedback. *Journal of Applied Sport Psychology, 22*(3), 247–261. doi:10.1080/10413201003666454

Elliot, D. L., Goldberg, L., Moe, E. L., Defrancesco, C. A., Durham, M. B., McGinnis, W., & Lockwood, C. (2008). Long-term outcomes of the ATHENA (Athletes Targeting Healthy Exercise & Nutrition Alternatives) program for female high school athletes. *Journal of Alcohol and Drug Education, 52*(2), 73–92.

Fearnow-Kenney, M., Wyrick, D. L., Milroy, J. J., Reifsteck, E. J., Day, T., & Kelly, S. E. (2016). The effects of a Web-based alcohol prevention program on social norms, expectancies, and intentions to prevent harm among college student-athletes. *The Sport Psychologist, 30*(2), 113–122. doi:10.1123/tsp.2015-0016

Gardner, F. L., & Moore, Z. E. (2007). *The psychology of enhancing human performance: The mindfulness-acceptance-commitment approach.* New York, NY: Springer.

Garmezy, N. (1993). Children in poverty: Resilience despite risk. *Psychiatry, 56*(1), 127–136. doi:10.1080/00332747.1993.11024627

Goddard, M. (2004). An assessment of the effectiveness of the CHAMPS /Life skills program at the university of north texas: A pilot study (Order No. 3126573). Available from ProQuest Dissertations & Theses Global (305167870). Retrieved from http://ezproxy.lib.utah.edu/docview/305167870?accountid=14677

Goldberg, L., Elliot, D., Clarke, G. N., MacKinnon, D. P., Moe, E., Zoref, L., ... Lapin, A. (1996). Effects of a multidimensional anabolic steroid prevention intervention: The Adolescents Training and Learning to Avoid Steroids (ATLAS) Program. *JAMA, 276,* 1555–1562. doi:10.1001/jama.1996.03540190027025

Goldberg, L., Elliot, D. L. (2005). Preventing substance use among high school athletes. *Journal of Applied School Psychology, 21*(2), 63–87. doi:10.1300/J370v21n02_05

Goldberg, L., Mackinnon, D., Elliot, D. L., Moe, E. L., Clarke, G., & Cheong, J. W. (2000). The Adolescents Training and Learning to Avoid Steroids program: Preventing drug use and promoting health behaviors. *Archives of Pediatrics and Adolescent Medicine, 154*(4), 332–338.

Gordon, R. (1987). An operational classification of disease prevention. In J. A. Steinberg & M. M. Silverman (Eds.), *Preventing mental disorders* (pp. 20–26). Rockville, MD: Department of Health and Human Services.

Hawkins, J. D., Catalano, R. F., & Miller, J. Y. (1992). Risk and protective factors for alcohol and other drug problems in adolescence and early adulthood: Implications for substance abuse prevention. *Psychological Bulletin, 112*(1), 64–105.

Ivarsson, A., Johnson, U., Andersen, M. B., Fallby, J., & Altemyr, M. (2015). It pays to pay attention: A mindfulness-based program for injury prevention with soccer players. *Journal of Applied Sport Psychology, 27*(3), 319–334. doi:10.1080/10413200.2015.1008072

Krawczynski, J. (2015). *NBA rookies learn about pitfalls in transition program.* Retrieved from http://www.nba.com/2015/news/08/13/nba-rookies-transition-program-karl-anthony-towns/

Kroshus, E., & DeFreese, J. D. (2017). Athlete burnout prevention strategies used by U.S. collegiate soccer coaches. *The Sport Psychologist, 31*(4), 332–343. doi:10.1123/tsp.2016-0067

Levi, J., Segal, L. M., & Juliano, C. (2008). *Prevention for a healthier America: Investments in disease prevention yield significant savings, stronger communities.* Retrieved from https://www.preventioninstitute.org/sites/default/files/publications/Prevention%20for%20a%20Healthier%20America_0.pdf

MacMullan, J. (2018). *The courageous fight to fix the NBA's mental health problem.* Retrieved from http://www.espn.com/nba/story/_/id/24382693/jackie-macmullan-kevin-love-paul-pierce-state-mental-health-nba

Martens, M. P., Kilmer, J. R., Beck, N. C., & Zamboanga, B. L. (2010). The efficacy of a targeted personalized drinking feedback intervention among intercollegiate athletes: A randomized controlled trial. *Psychology of Addictive Behaviors, 24*(4), 660–669. doi:10.1037/a0020299

Miller, P. S., & Kerr, G. A. (2002). Conceptualizing excellence: Past, present, and future. *Journal of Applied Sport Psychology, 14*(3), 140–153. doi:10.1080/10413200290103464

Morris, R. (1957). Prevention of chronic illness. *Social Work, 3*(2), 115. doi:10.1093/sw/3.2.115

National Collegiate Athletic Association. (n.d.). *Life skills.* Retrieved from http://www.ncaa.org/about/resources/leadership-development/life-skills

Perna, F. M., Antoni, M. H., Baum, A., Gordon, P., & Schneiderman, N. (2003). Cognitive behavioral stress management effects on injury and illness among competitive athletes: A randomized clinical trial. *Annals of Behavioral Medicine, 25*(1), 66–73. doi:10.1207/S15324796ABM2501_09

Ranby, K. W., Aiken, L. S., MacKinnon, D. P., Elliot, D. L., Moe, E. L., McGinnis, W., & Goldberg, L. (2009). A mediation analysis of the ATHENA Intervention for Female Athletes: Prevention of athletic-enhancing substance use and unhealthy weight loss behaviors. *Journal of Pediatric Psychology, 34*, 1069–1083. doi:10.1093/jpepsy/jsp025

Rosen, L., Manor, O., Engelhard, D., & Zucker, D. (2006). In defense of the randomized controlled trial for health promotion research. *American Journal of Public Health, 96*, 1181–1186.

Rumbold, J. L., Fletcher, D., & Daniels, K. (2012). A systematic review of stress management interventions with sport performers. *Sport, Exercise, and Performance Psychology, 1*(3), 173–193. doi:10.1037/a0026628

Smith, R. E. (1986). Toward a cognitive-affective model of athletic burnout. *Journal of Sport Psychology, 8*(1), 36–50. doi:10.1123/jsp.8.1.36

Starfield, B., Hyde, J., Gérvas, J., & Heath, I. (2008). The concept of prevention: A good idea gone astray? *Journal of Epidemiology & Community Health, 62*, 580–583.

SUNY Polytechnic Institute Athletics. (n.d.). *NCAA champs/life skills*. Retrieved from http://wildcats.sunypoly.edu/information/life_skills/index

Thombs, D. L., & Hamilton, M. J. (2002). Effects of a social norm feedback campaign on the drinking norms and behavior of Division I student-athletes. *Journal of Drug Education, 32*(3), 227–244. doi:10.2190/2UYU-6X9M-RJ65-3YYH

Tones, K. (2000). Evaluating health promotion: A tale of three errors. *Patient Education and Counseling, 39*(2–3), 227–236. doi:10.1016/S0738-3991(99)00035-X

U.S. Center for SafeSport. (2018). *Who we are: Collaborating to create a positive sport culture*. Retrieved from https://safesport.org/who-we-are

U.S. Department of Health and Human Services, Centers for Disease Control and Prevention, & Office of the Director, Office of Strategy and Innovation. (2011). *Introduction to program evaluation for public health programs: A self-study guide*. Atlanta, GA: Centers for Disease Control and Prevention. Retrieved from https://www.cdc.gov/eval/guide/cdcevalmanual.pdf

Voelker, D. K., & Petrie, T. A. (2017). *Bodies in motion: An evaluation of a program to support positive body image in female collegiate athletes*. Retrieved from https://www.ncaa.org/sites/default/files/2017RES_NCAAGrant-FinalReportExtension-VoelkerPetrie-FINAL_20171106.pdf

Weisz, J. R., Sandler, I. N., Durlak, J. A., & Anton, B. S. (2005). Promoting and protecting youth mental health through evidence-based prevention and treatment. *American Psychologist, 60*(6), 628–648. doi:10.1037/0003-066X.60.6.628

Wechsler, H., Davenport, A. E., Dowdall, G. W., Grossman, S. J., & Zanakos, S. I. (1997). Binge drinking, tobacco, and illicit drug use and involvement in college athletics. *Journal of American College Health, 45*(5), 195–200. doi:10.1080/07448481.1997.9936884

Woolf, S. H., Husten, C. G., Lewin, L. S., Marks, J. S., Fielding, J. E., & Sanchez, E. J. (2009). *The economic argument for disease prevention: Distinguishing between value and savings*. Retrieved from http://prevent.org/data/files/initiatives/economicargumentfordiseaseprevention.pdf

10

ORGANIZATIONAL PRACTICES AND POLICY

Administrators of a high-level ice hockey league have recently become aware of abusive behavior by several coaches in the league. The reports include accusations of both physical and emotional abuse during practices. Concerned about the safety and well-being of the players, and following meetings with several key stakeholders (e.g., league sponsors, players, coaches, team staff), the administrators decide that there is a need to create league-wide standards for coach conduct, including expectations, guidelines for reporting, and repercussions for offenders. Unsure of how to properly design, implement, and evaluate policy, the league hires an outside consultant with experience in public health policy. Following a thorough needs assessment, the consultant recommends a multi-level approach to prevent future instances of coach misconduct, including education for coaches on how to effectively motivate and communicate with players, education for staff on recognizing abusive behavior, partnerships with local mental health professionals, and a clear code of conduct for coach behavior with associated consequences for violations. Although league administrators are pleased with the plan, the consultant stresses the importance of evaluating the policy and using these results to improve the content, implementation, and impact of the policy.

In the previous chapter I made a case for the importance of early intervention (i.e., health promotion, universal and selective prevention) to mitigate the effect of envirosocial threats to athletes' psychosocial health. Although intentionally planned, implemented, and evaluated prevention programs are an essential part of enhancing athlete well-being, such initiatives will only be as effective as the larger context allows them to be. That is, no matter the strength of a given prevention program, if athletes continue to perform in an environment that at best fails to reinforce, and at worst contradicts program content, meaningful change cannot be expected. In this chapter I propose changes to organizational practice and policy in sport as the gold standard for promoting positive psychosocial health in high-level athletes, and offer examples of sport policy in practice.

Policy as the cornerstone of comprehensive prevention practices

Policy refers broadly to a course of action used to guide decision-making (policy, n.d.). The World Health Organization notes that health-related policy serves to define a vision for the future, outline priorities, and build consensus (World Health Organization, 2018). Perhaps because it connotes politics, negotiation, and protracted efforts to successfully implement, the word "policy" is likely to elicit a cringe from athletes, coaches, and sport personnel. However, changes to policy and organizational practices have a long history of success in public health. For example, following the passing of a no-smoking law in restaurants and workplaces in Olmstead County, Minnesota, the number of heart attacks over the next 18 months dropped by 33% (Hurt et al., 2012).

Policy is one type of *primordial prevention*, which refers to measures taken to prevent the emergence of environmental, social, and behavioral conditions known to increase the risk of disease (Bonita, Beaglehole, & Kjellstrom, 2006; Strasser, 1978). As opposed to other forms of prevention discussed in Chapter 9, which work to reduce existing risk factors (e.g., lack of knowledge), the goal of primordial prevention is to make healthy behaviors the easy choice, and in doing so create societal norms that are supportive of such behaviors. Policy and legislation are at the forefront of a comprehensive approach to prevention which emphasizes the need for strategies that target environmental as well as individual factors. In the realm of high-level sport, policy creation was addressed in interviews with NCAA stakeholders (i.e., parents, coaches, and administrators) on parental involvement in student-athletes' sport experience (Kaye, Lowe, & Dorsch, 2018). Participants noted several elements of ideal policies governing parental involvement, including student-athlete empowerment, protecting sport as the coach's domain, communication with parents, building an understanding of the transition into college sport, facilitating parent-athlete communication, and parental education. Of course, as with any policy, stakeholders expressed several potential barriers and points to consider in advance of implementation, including potential lack of congruence between educational programming and university views on parental-involvement, feasibility, timing, and funding (or lack thereof). The barriers noted by stakeholders highlight how even policies based on sound evidence and with the best of intentions can be stifled by the bureaucracy of large organizations such as the NCAA.

The spectrum of prevention

Within the field of public health, Cohen's Spectrum of Prevention (Cohen & Swift, 1999) is one example of a comprehensive, multi-level, and interconnected perspective on prevention (see Figure 10.1). The spectrum depicts several distinct yet complementary types of prevention practices typically addressed in comprehensive prevention initiatives. Before elaborating on the role of policy in athlete psychosocial health, I first describe the lower-level prevention practices which can be supported by strong policy initiatives.

At the bottom of the spectrum are prevention practices aimed at enhancing individuals' knowledge and skills. Most of the prevention programs discussed in Chapter 9 exemplify a knowledge- and skill-building approach (e.g., stress management, awareness of challenges associated with transition). Because prevention targeting knowledge and skills tend to affect a relatively small number of individuals, it represents the smallest portion of the inverted triangle. Just above knowledge and skill building is health messaging, which consists of mass communication efforts designed to reach as many individuals as possible with targeted health-promoting messages. Within high-level sport, health messaging

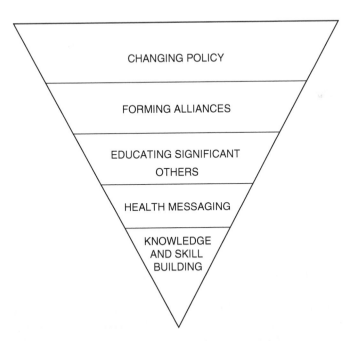

FIGURE 10.1 A model for comprehensive prevention practices in high-level sport. Adapted from Cohen, L., & Chehimi, S. (2010). The imperative for primary prevention. In L. Cohen, V. Chavez, & S. Chehimi (Eds.), *Prevention is primary: Strategies for community well-being* (p. 17). San Francisco, CA: Jossey-Bass

may occur through social media campaigns encouraging life-sport balance and healthy relationships.

Educating significant others is the next level of the spectrum, which is characterized by a "train-the-trainer" approach to prevention. In the sport context, anyone who works with and supports athletes on a day-to-day basis, including parents, coaches, athletic trainers, and administrative personnel, is considered a "significant other." Because these individuals are embedded in the lives of high-level athletes, educating them on the optimal type and timing of health-promoting messages, best practices for social support provision, and recognition of the signs and symptoms of athlete distress is an effective way to reinforce formal prevention programming. The next level of the spectrum involves forming alliances. Because the combined forces of multiple individuals and/or organizations sharing a common goal is more powerful than any single entity, alliances are commonplace in the field of public health. For example, the Centers for Disease Control and Prevention (CDC) Coalition includes over 100 organizations throughout the U.S. who work together to promote federal funding for health promotion programs and ensure that such programs are evidence-based (CDC, n.d.).

One of the major tasks of alliances is for members to work together to influence changes to the practices of individual organizations, as well as more wide-ranging policy and legislation supporting alliance priorities. A recent example of alliance-forming in high-level sport is the Player's Coalition, a group of current NFL players and team owners who have joined together to promote social change in the form of police and community relations, criminal justice reform, and education and economic advancement for low-income families (Player's Coalition, 2018). The Australian Athletes' Alliance (AAA) is another prominent alliance dedicated to elite athlete well-being. The eight elite sport associations comprising the AAA collaborate to promote strong governance, integrity, athlete development and well-being, and health and safety of elite Australian athletes (AAA, n.d.). I discuss the specific policies of AAA later in this chapter.

The subordinate levels of the spectrum are much likelier to succeed when governed by strong policies supporting healthy norms. The National College Players Association (NCPA) is one example of a sport alliance that has made contributions to health-promoting policies for athletes. Formed in 2001, the NCPA has spearheaded several NCAA policy changes resulting in enhanced legal protection, health, and safety of NCAA athletes (NCPA, 2017). According to their website, a few of the notable policy changes that the NCPA has championed include the elimination of healthcare restrictions for college athletes, new safety rules to prevent player injury/illness during practice, and the expansion of catastrophic-injury benefits (NCPA Victories, 2017). In countries where high-level sport is overseen by the federal government, more sweeping policy change is possible. The United Kingdom's Sporting Future is one such example. First published in December 2015, Sporting Future is a comprehensive plan for promoting all levels of sport and physical activity as a mechanism for well-being as well as personal, social, community, and economic development (Department for Digital, Culture, Media & Sport, 2015). Most relevant for the current text is the government's focus on emotional health for elite performers. The Mental Health and Elite Sport Action Plan (Department for Digital, Culture, Media & Sport, 2018) details six actions and associated outputs to be implemented across several years in support of elite athlete emotional health. The plan exemplifies a comprehensive and interconnected approach to prevention of emotional health concerns in elite UK athletes.

When viewed from the lens of the spectrum, the action plan itself is an example of overarching *policy* influencing all elite athletes in the UK. The action plan was made possible through the cooperative efforts of several UK organizations such as UK Sport, UK Coaching, and Mind, who formed an *alliance* dedicated to improving athletes' emotional health. One of the outputs targeted by the plan is training for sport personnel and *significant others* on how to recognize emotional health problems. Campaigns to promote awareness of support and reduce emotional health stigma represent a *health messaging* approach to prevention. Finally, the plan includes various *education and skill-building* opportunities for athletes, including information on the role of sport and clinical psychologists in promoting emotional health, and support for the transition out of elite sport. In sum, the UK's Mental Health and Elite Sport Action Plan is a prime example of a comprehensive, multi-level, and interconnected approach to prevention in high-level sport. In the remaining sections I highlight some other policy initiatives aimed at minimizing the effect of the threats discussed in Chapters 4–8, and promoting psychosocial health in high-level athletes.

USOC athlete safety policy

To ensure a safe and positive training environment for all U.S. athletes, in 2018 the USOC adopted the Athlete Safety Policy (Team USA, 2018). The policy applies to all USOC employees, coaches, athletes, and staff, and details prohibited behaviors (e.g., bullying, hazing, harassment, sexual misconduct), as well as the protocol for reporting such behaviors. Further included in the written policy are investigation and resolution procedures (e.g., hearing process, appropriate sanctions), which are handled by the U.S. Center for SafeSport. The final portion of the policy emphasizes mandatory SafeSport Awareness Training, discussed in Chapter 9, for all USOC employees, including those employed by national governing bodies (NGBs). Because the Athlete Safety Policy is new, data regarding its effectiveness in reducing reports of misconduct and abuse are so far unavailable. Such evaluation data will provide important feedback on whether the policy has had its intended effect on athlete safety, and/or requires revision.

AAA policy platform

As previously discussed, the AAA works to promote the well-being of both the institution of elite sport and the athletes who compete within this system in

Australia. Their Policy Platform document details the four policies and associated strategies advocated by the AAA (AAA, n.d.). Two of the four policies—Athlete Development and Well-Being, and Health & Safety—are particularly relevant for athletes' psychosocial health. Among the actions taken in support of the aforementioned policies are the development of personalized player-development action plans, access to counseling for athletes, education and preparation for transition out of sport, an annual conference supporting athlete development, advocacy for competition schedules that maintain athlete well-being, and advocacy for the adoption of mental-health programs for athletes. An important inclusion in the AAA's platform is an explicit emphasis on social well-being, which is particularly evident within the policy focused on athlete development and well-being. Specifically, the AAA seeks to empower athletes by arming them with knowledge and skills, protect them from discrimination by advocating for training environments free of discrimination and abuse, and promote holistic well-being by prioritizing sport-life balance.

U.S. Figure Skating policy on athlete health and well-being

As discussed in Chapters 2 and 6, the pressure to perform at a high level can sometimes influence athletes to engage in unhealthy behaviors. Chief among such behaviors, especially in sports focused on leanness and aesthetics, are those aimed at altering body weight, shape, and size (Voelker & Galli, in press). Figure skating is one example of a sport where athletes often face intense pressure from coaches, judges, and other skaters to "slim down" for both appearance and performance, which can lead to pathological body-modification strategies (Voelker, Gould, & Reel, 2014). As a result, U.S. Figure Skating (USFS, 2011) published a 20-page document detailing their position on matters of appearance, weight management, and eating behaviors in U.S. figure skaters.

The underlying message of the USFS policy statement is that athlete health and well-being should take priority over appearance and performance. The document includes narratives addressing the unique role played by coaches, officials, family/friends, and athletes themselves in promoting healthy eating, weight management, and body image (U.S. Figure Skating 2011). To this end, the document lists three broad actions to be employed: (a) education for all U.S. Figure Skating (USFS) members, (b) development of policy addressing risk factors for disordered eating and eating disorders, and (c) establishing links to treatment resources. Presumably because they are the individuals with the most power over skaters, USFS focuses their policies solely on coaches' and officials' weight- and appearance-based communication with skaters. Of note are guidelines related to weighing, language/word choice, and conversations regarding body weight or appearance. For example, the document states that "A coach should only weigh an athlete with a specific cause and use the utmost sensitivity and confidentiality" (U.S. Figure Skating 2011, p. 5). Another coach-directed guideline states that "Language/word choice has impact. Use words sensitively and non-judgmentally. Focus on performance and fitness rather than appearance and body weight" (U.S. Figure Skating 2011, p. 5). USFS prohibits officials from discussing an individual's weight or body composition independent of performance or elements of skaters' non-bodily appearance (e.g., costume, makeup). The USFS policy appears useful in terms of promoting a healthier culture around body weight and appearance for U.S. figure skaters. However, the document lacks any mention of enforcement or repercussions for violation of the policy, which are integral for long-term success (Cohen & Chehimi, 2010). Further, the policy document was published several years ago, but as with other prevention practices discussed in Chapters 9 and 10, it appears that there has been no attempt at evaluating its success.

Conclusion

Because of its capacity to produce widespread changes to the norms and culture of an organization, policy represents the most powerful means of promoting psychosocial health and well-being in high-level athletes. Within public health, policy is the cornerstone of comprehensive prevention, and has contributed to reductions in illness and mortality related to factors such as sanitation, tobacco, and motor vehicle crashes (CDC, 2011). As awareness of threats to athlete psychosocial health grows, several high-level sport organizations have enacted their own policies to prevent psychosocial health concerns and promote athlete well-being. In this chapter I highlighted several such policies, ranging from those which consist of a series of guidelines (e.g., USFS Athlete Well-being), to those taking a more comprehensive approach by integrating policy with specific prevention programming, coach/staff education, and health messaging campaigns (e.g., the UK's Mental Health and Elite Athlete Action Plan).

Although most policies adopted by high-level sport groups seem logical, little information is available on the planning process leading to policy development and implementation. For example, a standard procedure for the adoption of most public health policies is a thorough needs assessment of the assets and challenges of a given community (Themba-Nixon, 2010). Themba-Nixon offered a multi-step process for policy formation that includes consideration of community/organizational needs, use of strategies such as media advocacy to garner support, and eventual enforcement of the policy. Although the policies of sport governing bodies may not require all the same steps as those used for the general population, some form of due diligence seems necessary to ensure desired results. Unfortunately, the sponsoring organizations for the policies discussed in this chapter fail to offer much, if any, insight on the process used to arrive at their final policies. Such information is important, as policies based on well-conducted needs assessments are likely to be much more effective in achieving long-term goals compared to policies arising from "knee-jerk" reactions to adverse events and associated negative media coverage.

A second, related weakness of policies focused on athlete health and well-being is an apparent lack of evaluation by most organizations. Other than the UK's action plan, which contained relatively detailed outputs and timelines for each policy activity, there is an alarming lack of concern from sport organizations with measuring whether policies have had or will have their desired effect. Although the process of policy evaluation can be costly in terms of both time and money, it is a necessary step in ensuring the fidelity and utility of a given policy. The CDC's National Center for Injury Prevention and Control (n.d.) suggests that policies be evaluated at three levels: (a) content (i.e., does the policy document align with the underlying goals and logic of the policy?), (b) implementation (i.e., was the policy employed as intended?), and (c) impact (i.e., did the policy influence change in pre-determined outcomes?). For example, the USOC would be wise to evaluate the implementation and impact of their Athlete Safety Policy. Specifically, are the procedures for reporting abuse being followed as directed? And even if so, has the policy increased athletes' and staff members' knowledge of abuse? More importantly, has the policy contributed to a decrease in the number of reported cases of abuse and misconduct within U.S. sport? Given the large amount of resources often devoted to the implementation of sport policies, it seems critical for administrators to know whether these resources are well spent, or whether they may be better spent in other ways.

References

Australian Athletes' Alliance. (n.d.). *What we stand for.* Retrieved from https://www.ausathletesall.com.au/what-we-stand-for

Bonita, R. Beaglehole, R., & Kjellström, T. (2006). *Basic epidemiology* (2nd ed.). World Health Organization. Retrieved from whqlibdoc.who.int/publications/2006/9241547073_eng.pdf 2006

Centers for Disease Control and Prevention. (2011). *Ten great public health achievements—United States, 2001–2010.* Retrieved from https://www.cdc.gov/mmwr/preview/mmwrhtml/mm6019a5.htm

Centers for Disease Control and Prevention. (n.d.). *CDC Coalition.* Retrieved from http://www.cdccoalition.org/

Centers for Disease Control and Prevention National Center for Injury Prevention and Control. (n.d.). *Step by step—Evaluating violence and injury prevention policies. Brief 1: Overview of policy evaluation.* Retrieved from https://www.cdc.gov/injury/pdfs/policy/Brief%201-a.pdf

Cohen, L., & Chehimi, S. (2010). The imperative for primary prevention. In L. Cohen, V. Chavez, & S. Chehimi (Eds.), *Prevention is primary: Strategies for community well-being.* San Francisco, CA: Jossey-Bass.

Cohen, L., & Swift, S. (1999). The spectrum of prevention: Developing a comprehensive approach to injury prevention. *Injury Prevention, 9*(5), 203–207.

Department for Digital, Culture, Media & Sport. (2015, December 17). *Sporting Future—A new strategy for an active nation.* Retrieved from https://www.gov.uk/government/publications/sporting-future-a-new-strategy-for-an-active-nation

Department for Digital, Culture, Media & Sport. (2018, March 21). *Mental health and elite sport action plan.* Retrieved from https://www.gov.uk/government/publications/mental-health-and-elite-sport-action-plan

Hurt, R. D., Weston, S. A., Ebbert, J. O., McNallan, S. M., Croghan, I. T., Schroeder, D. R., & Roger, V. L. (2012). Myocardial infarction and sudden cardiac death in Olmsted County, Minnesota, before and after smoke-free workplace laws. *Archives of Internal Medicine, 172*(21), 1635-41. doi:10.1001/2013.jamainternmed.46

Kaye, M. P., Lowe, K., & Dorsch, T. E. (2018). Dyadic examination of parental support, basic needs satisfaction, and student-athlete development during emerging adulthood. *Journal of Family Issues.* doi:10.1177/0192513X18806557

National College Players Association. (2017). *NCPA victories.* Retrieved from https://www.ncpanow.org/ncpa-victories

Player's Coalition. (2018, September 5). *The fight continues.* Retrieved from https://www.theplayerstribune.com/en-us/articles/football-players-coalition-the-fight-continues

policy. (2018) In *Merriam-Webster.* Retrieved from https://www.merriam-webster.com/dictionary/policy

Strasser, T. (1978). Reflections on cardiovascular diseases. *Interdisciplinary Science Reviews, 3*(3), 225–230. doi:10.1179/030801878791925921

Team USA. (2018). *Safe sport.* Retrieved from https://www.teamusa.org/Home/Team%20USA%20Athlete%20Services/Safe%20Sport

Themba-Nixon, M. (2010). The power of local communities to foster policy. In L. Cohen, V. Chavez, & S. Chehimi (Eds.), *Prevention is primary: Strategies for community well-being* (2nd ed.). San Francisco, CA: Jossey-Bass.

U.S. Figure Skating. (2011). *U.S. Figure Skating policy on athlete health and well-being: Appearance, weight management, disordered eating and eating disorders.* Retrieved from https://www.usfigureskating.org/content/Nutrition%20position%20paper%20Aug%202011.pdf

Voelker, D. K., & Galli, N. (in press). *APA handbook of sport and exercise psychology.* Washington, DC: American Psychological Association.

Voelker, D. K., Gould, D., & Reel, J. J. (2014). Prevalence and correlates of disordered eating in female figure skaters. *Psychology of Sport and Exercise, 15,* 696–704. doi:10.1016/j.psychsport.2013.12.002

World Health Organization. (2018). *Health policy.* Retrieved from http://www.who.int/topics/health_policy/en/

11

TREATMENT

Jayson is a 23-year-old professional baseball player, who after five seasons has worked his way to the major league team. Team staff think highly of Jayson's skills, and expect him to be a solid contributor to the team. However, they do have some concerns about his behavior toward teammates and the media. Always viewed as a bit aloof, Jayson has become even more so in recent months. He isolates himself from teammates in the clubhouse, actively avoids reporters after games, and is noticeably uncomfortable in even the most benign social situations. His teammates describe him as being awkward, and are unsure of how to approach him. After a conversation with management, Jayson agrees to meet with the team's psychologist. Based upon an intake session, the psychologist diagnoses Jayson with social anxiety disorder, and recommends several sessions of cognitive behavioral therapy, along with a referral to a psychiatrist for possible prescription of an anti-anxiety medication. After several weeks, although Jayson is still by no means a social butterfly, he appears much more relaxed around his team. He reports that both the medication and therapy have enabled him to better cope with uncomfortable social situations.

Although strong prevention efforts can reduce incidents of psychosocial health problems (Saxena, Jané-Llopis, & Hosman, 2006), and in some cases reduce costs (e.g., Wellander, Wells, & Feldman, 2016), complete prevention is unlikely. When psychosocial health concerns do manifest, treatment, also known as tertiary prevention, becomes the priority. In recent years, several high-level athletes have sought the use of mental health counseling for issues such as anxiety, depression, and substance abuse, and advocated for greater acceptance of these conditions in the sporting realm (Gleeson & Brady, 2017). Prominent athletes such as basketball player Kevin Love, American gymnast Simone Biles, and American football player Brandon Marshall have been at the forefront of criticizing traditional views of psychosocial health concerns as a sign of mental weakness, and de-stigmatizing common psychosocial disorders (Boren, 2018; Cogan, 2014). In this chapter I present an overview of psychosocial health treatment for high-level athletes. First, I discuss the various forms that treatment may take, and their efficacy. Second, I highlight the unique barriers to treatment for high-level athletes. Finally, I offer an overview of the state of psychosocial treatment services for high-level athletes in various sport organizations.

Forms of psychosocial treatment for athletes

The National Alliance on Mental Illness (NAMI) lists common types of psychosocial treatment, several of which have relevance for athletes (NAMI, 2018). In the following sections I focus on two forms of treatment and their application in high-level sport: (a) psychotherapy, and (b) psychoeducation. Although psychotropic medications are often part of the treatment plan for individuals with psychosocial health conditions, a focus on these drugs is beyond the scope of this text. I instead refer interested readers to Reardon and Factor (2010) for further information on the use of psychiatric medications for treating psychosocial health problems in athletes.

Psychotherapy

One of the most common forms of treatment for psychosocial concerns is *psychotherapy*. Psychotherapy occurs when individuals work with trained therapists/ mental health counselors to overcome or manage their psychosocial health problems (Herkov, 2016). Psychotherapists attempt to promote positive change in clients by establishing a therapeutic relationship (aka the *therapeutic alliance*) and using effective communication practices to help individuals gain self-awareness and learn strategies for handling challenging situations (Herkov, 2016). Although therapists may choose from a variety of therapeutic approaches in their work with athletes (e.g., psychoanalysis, behavior therapy), cognitive behavioral therapies (CBT) such as Albert Ellis' (1957) rational emotive behavior therapy (REBT), and Beck's (1970) cognitive therapy are among the most commonly used for both emotional health and sport performance enhancement. The popularity of CBT in sport stems from several factors, including their time-limited nature, an emphasis on empowering athletes to take control of their thoughts, and a substantial body of evidence supporting their effectiveness for ameliorating conditions such as depression, anxiety, and eating disorders in the general population (e.g., David, Cotet, Matu, Mogoase, & Stefan, 2018; Linardon, 2018).

Further, athletes are likely to find some comfort in CBT-based therapy, which in some ways mirrors the structure and prescribed repetition associated with sport training (Hays, 1999). Within sport, CBT-based interventions have been used to help athletes manage unhealthy perfectionism (Gustaffson & Lundqvist, 2016), ease post-concussive symptoms (Splete, 2016), reduce performance anxiety (Gustaffson, Lundqvist, & Tod, 2017), optimize appraisals of organizational stressors (Didymus & Fletcher, 2017), and help athletes cope with injury (Mahoney & Hanrahan, 2011).

REBT-based techniques focused on reducing irrational beliefs (e.g., "I must *always* do well," "Others must *always* treat me nicely.") and promoting more functional patterns of thinking/self-talk are often employed by sport psychologists focused on performance enhancement (e.g., Vealey, 2005). Despite being the oldest form of CBT, it was not until recently that researchers took an interest in testing the effectiveness of REBT on indicators of psychosocial health in athletes. Turner et al. (e.g., Cunningham & Turner, 2016; Turner & Barker, 2013) have conducted and evaluated numerous REBT interventions with athletes. Interventions included face-to-face sessions in which athletes learned the fundamentals of REBT and had the opportunity to apply these principles to themselves. In one study, players at an elite youth soccer academy attended a single 60-minute workshop in which they were taught strategies for recognizing and disputing irrational beliefs. Although players' endorsement of irrational beliefs decreased immediately following the workshop, they returned to pre-workshop levels six weeks later.

Recognizing the limitations of the one-time group session approach, Deen, Turner, and Wong (2017) conducted a series of five, 60-minute, one-on-one REBT sessions with five elite squash players. In addition, players completed homework to reinforce the in-session content. A key aim of the intervention was to promote rational beliefs through the development of personal credos prompting athletes to think rationally about various circumstances they would encounter. Not only did all athletes report a decrease in irrational beliefs, but three of the five also reported an increase in self-reported resilient qualities (Deen et al., 2017). In another study, mixed martial arts fighters exposed to REBT reported reduced irrationality and self-depreciation and increased unconditional self-acceptance. Most importantly, these changes remained in two of the three athletes 6 months post-intervention. Thus, REBT shows some promise for enhancing psychosocial health in non-clinical high-level athletes. A logical next step is to test REBT as a psychotherapeutic treatment for athletes with diagnosed psychosocial health problems such as anxiety, depression, and eating disorders.

As principles of mindfulness, such as present moment contact and non-judgmental awareness, have been embraced by sport psychology practitioners for performance enhancement (e.g., Bühlmayer, Birrer, Röthlin, Faude, & Donath, 2017), there is similar interest in applying mindfulness-focused CBT approaches (e.g., acceptance and commitment therapy) for enhancing athletes' psychosocial health and well-being. Mahoney and Hanrahan (2011) implemented a

four-session, one-on-one acceptance and commitment therapy (ACT) intervention with four injured athletes. Athletes were educated on several key elements
of ACT, including cognitive defusion, mindfulness, acceptance, and values, and
the researchers guided athletes through experiential exercises to reinforce each
element. Although little quantitative change in athletes' self-reported mindfulness, injury anxiety, and acceptance was noted from pre- to post-intervention, in
post-intervention interviews the athletes reported that they found several of the
techniques useful, and would use them again in the future.

Influenced by the shift from thought-control-focused CBT approaches to
mindfulness-based approaches in clinical and counseling psychology, Gardner
and Moore (2004) introduced a sport-specific model of performance and well-
being enhancement for athletes—the mindfulness-acceptance-commitment
program (MAC). MAC is a seven-module program aimed at promoting mindful awareness and non-judgmental acceptance in athletes (Gardner & Moore,
2004). Although primarily used as an approach for performance enhancement,
Gross, Moore, Gardner, Wolanin, Pess, and Marks (2018) recently examined
the psychosocial health benefits of MAC. Using a sample of female collegiate
athletes, the researchers compared pre-post changes in self-reported psychological distress, psychological flexibility, emotion regulation, and mindful awareness
between randomly assigned groups of 11 student-athletes receiving the seven-
week MAC program and 11 student-athletes receiving a seven-week psychological skills training program. As hypothesized, the athletes receiving the MAC
intervention reported positive changes in psychological distress, substance abuse,
and hostility. Further, athletes who received the MAC intervention reported
significant decreases in general anxiety, disordered eating, and distress between
the end of the intervention and the one-month follow-up. The athletes receiving
psychological skills training did not report any significant changes in the psychosocial health variables. Because of its sport-specific approach, the MAC protocol
holds promise as a psychosocial health treatment approach in high-level athletes.
The authors also suggested that MAC may be used as a tool for primary prevention in athletes, and this represents a fruitful line of investigation for the future.

Psychoeducation and support groups

The first module of the MAC protocol, psychoeducation, is also another common form of psychosocial treatment. *Psychoeducation* involves educating individuals about a health condition that they or their loved ones are experiencing
(Virtual Medical Centre, 2014). The health condition addressed in psychoeducation may or may not be of a psychosocial nature, but the goal is always to
use education of the physical, psychological, and social factors associated with
the health condition as a way of alleviating distress and enhancing self-efficacy
(Virtual Medical Centre, 2014). Because groups offer potential for individuals to
positively influence each other through factors such as the instillation of hope,
imparting of information, and conveying the feeling that they are not alone in

their experiences (Yalom, 1995), psychoeducation, often, but not always, occurs in a group setting (Gerrity & De-Lucia-Waack, 2006).

Within sport, the health condition targeted may be any of the threats discussed in this text, including transition, injury, or organizational stress. Alternatively, psychoeducation may be employed to address maladaptive patterns of thinking, such as was done by Mosewich, Crocker, Kowalski, and DeLongis (2013) in evaluating a psychoeducational self-compassion intervention with female collegiate athletes. Danish, Petitpas, and Hale (1993) made a case for the power of psychoeducation to enhance athletes' life skills and promote healthy behaviors. The authors discussed a psychoeducational program known as Going for the Goal (Goal), in which student-athletes learned to set goals and develop action plans for attaining them, including strategies for handling barriers and proper use of social support. Although the authors reported positive feedback from participants, no formal evaluation data was presented.

Psychoeducation with athletes has most often been used to support the process of transition. For example, freshman collegiate student-athletes who participated in an eight-session program of psychoeducation regarding the transition into college sport reported the experience as helpful for managing transition stress, and strongly recommended the program to future students (Harris, Alterkuse, & Engels, 2003). In another study, female collegiate athletes reported being satisfied with a retirement transition program that included psychoeducation (Constantine, 1995). Unfortunately, researchers have not included control groups when examining the effectiveness of psychoeducation on adjustment to transition. Nor have they assessed the influence of psychoeducational programs on psychological and subjective well-being (e.g., life purpose, life satisfaction, affect).

Unique barriers to psychosocial treatment in high-level athletes

Despite progress in the awareness of and action toward the treatment of psychosocial health concerns in athletes, many challenges remain. Chief among these challenges is the stigma around emotional health concerns and help-seeking that continues to exist in the high-level sport environment (Moreland, Coxe, & Yang, 2018). Wahto, Swift, and Whipple (2016) conducted an important study on the role of stigma in predicting college student-athletes' attitudes toward psychosocial help-seeking. The researchers considered the influence of both *self-stigma*, or negative attitudes toward oneself for engaging in a given behavior, and *public-stigma*, or the perceptions of negative attitudes that others may have about one's behavior, on 43 collegiate student-athletes' attitudes toward seeking mental health services (Wahto et al., 2016). After controlling for gender and treatment history, the two stigma variables accounted for a robust 66% of the variance in help-seeking attitudes. Athletes reported being more willing to seek help when referred by a family member as compared to a coach, teammate, or when considering seeking help on their own.

So, although the public disclosure of psychosocial health concerns by high-profile athletes has likely resulted in some help-seeking de-stigmatization, the findings of Wahto et al. (2016) suggest that stigma is still a powerful barrier preventing athletes from acting on psychosocial health concerns. And despite the finding of no significant gender difference in help-seeking by Wahto et al., several researchers have found that male athletes, and especially those who have internalized a hyper-masculine identity, are significantly less likely to seek treatment for psychosocial health issues (e.g., M. Steinfeldt & J. A. Steinfeldt, 2012). The reticence of male athletes to seek treatment is not surprising, as men in the general population are more deterred by stigma than women (Clement et al., 2015), and the hyper-masculine nature of certain sports likely heightens male athletes' sense that psychosocial health concerns are a sign of mental weakness (M. Steinfeldt & J. A. Steinfeldt, 2012).

Although stigma may represent the most powerful barrier to psychosocial health treatment in athletes, sport psychiatrists have identified several other factors that make treatment of this population uniquely challenging (Stillman, Brown, Ritvo, & Glick, 2016). First, the training demands of high-level sport can result in symptoms which mimic those of clinical disorders (e.g., burnout vs. clinical depression). Second, Stillman et al. (2016) noted how some athletes engage in rigid and ritualistic behaviors that can be confused with obsessive compulsive disorder. Third, when athletes perceive that a certain behavior, such as disordered eating or performance enhancing substance use, confers a performance advantage, they may be reluctant to engage in a process aimed at changing these practices. Finally, the social stature afforded to some high-level athletes may result in a sense of entitlement, in which athletes expect special accommodations related to the timing and location of sessions (Stillman et al., 2016). Thus, clinicians who provide psychosocial treatment to high-level athletes need to be especially mindful of balancing the unique needs of these individuals with the delivery of ethical and quality care.

The current state of psychosocial health treatment services for high-level athletes

The last decade has seen a growing concern for athlete psychosocial health by high-level sport organizations (Kliegman, 2017). In the U.S., the NCAA has been at the forefront in promoting research and practice related to optimizing student-athletes' emotional health. Since the inception of the Sport Science Institute in 2013, the NCAA has awarded research grants for psychosocial-based intervention projects and published a variety of resources for athletes and those with a vested interest in student-athlete psychosocial health (NCAA, n.d.). Although the total number of professionals dealing with psychosocial health at NCAA member institutions remains elusive, it has likely grown from the fewer than 25 full-time professionals employed in 2014 (Noren, 2014). Of course, it is also likely that many of the over 1,200 NCAA institutions, and particularly those at the Division II and III levels, lack a full-time mental health professional. Although many collegiate athletics departments partner with the on-campus university counseling center to support student-athletes treatment needs, the presence of a dedicated psychologist or other mental health practitioner enhances the probability that athletes and coaches will seek help (Kliegman, 2017). Even at those institutions with a full-time position, it is doubtful that one person can adequately address the psychosocial health needs of several hundred student-athletes. Some athletics departments have begun using post-doctoral clinical or counseling psychology student interns to enhance quality of care (e.g., USC Student Health, n.d.). However, given that there are almost 500,000 student-athletes across North America, the NCAA must remain committed to supporting member institutions in improving the staff-to-athlete ratio for psychosocial healthcare.

Similar to the NCAA, other high-level sport organizations have displayed support for psychosocial health services for athletes. Although decisions regarding psychosocial health services are at the professional level are at the discretion of individual clubs/teams, organization administrators and players' unions have a large role in advocating for the psychosocial health needs of athletes. Several major professional sport leagues have done just that in recent years. In 2012, the Professional Footballers' Association, which is the labor union for professional footballers in England and Wales, began assisting current and former players in obtaining treatment for emotional health concerns (Keble, 2016). As of 2014, all 20 clubs in the English Premier League had a full-time mental health professional on staff (Hughes, 2014). In the National Basketball Association, the league and players' association have partnered to provide players with emotional health resources (Reynolds, 2018). Of all professional sport organizations, however, the National Football League (NFL) appears to offer the most comprehensive psychosocial treatment services to its athletes. All NFL players participate in the league's Total Wellness program, which includes mandatory psychoeducation for rookies on a variety of psychosocial health topics (e.g., stress management, relationships, decision-making), as well as a service called *Life Line*, which is a confidential 24/7 phone line for current and former NFL players, coaches, or staff dealing with an emotional health crisis (Rapaport, 2012). Further, all NFL players receive eight free counseling sessions for themselves or any member of their household. An additional strength of Total Wellness is its *train-the-trainer* approach, in which former NFL players are used as transition coaches for retiring players, and team staff are trained to recognize and appropriately handle emotional health crises (Clay, 2017). Although no data are publicly available on the number of players who have taken advantage of these services, or the effect of the program on relevant long-term health outcomes, the NFL's multifaceted approach appears to have promise for both the treatment and prevention of psychosocial health concerns in its players.

Conclusion

Although primary prevention should remain a priority for high-level sport organizations, the strong demands on athletes require that organizations are ready to support those who do need psychosocial treatment. CBT-oriented psychotherapy and psychoeducation are common modalities of treatment for high-level athletes. However, a lack of rigorous evaluation, particularly regarding psychoeducation, precludes a complete understanding of what works best for athletes. Further, despite calls for the use of psychoeducation with injured athletes (e.g., Naylor, Clement, Shannon, & Connole, 2011; Granito, Hogan, & Varnum, 1995), no researchers have undertaken an evaluation of such a program. Even if certain treatments are found to be effective, challenges remain in the provision of psychosocial health services to athletes. Such challenges include self and public stigma around help-seeking (particularly for male athletes), the overlap of certain clinical disorders with typical athlete behaviors, and issues of entitlement for certain high-profile athletes. Public disclosure of psychosocial health struggles by several high-profile athletes has prompted sport governing bodies such as the NCAA, English Premier League, NBA, and NFL to invest in treatment-based initiatives. As discussed regarding prevention in Chapters 9 and 10, organization-sponsored psychosocial treatment efforts await proper evaluation of both the process and the impact of these services.

References

Beck, A. T. (1970). Cognitive therapy: Nature and relation to behavior therapy. *Behavior Therapy, 1*(2), 184–200. doi:10.1016/S0005-7894(70)80030-2

Boren, C. (2018, March 6). "Everything was spinning": Kevin Love opens up about his in-game panic attack. *Washington Post*. Retrieved from https://www.washingtonpost.com/news/early-lead/wp/2018/03/06/everything-was-spinning-kevin-love-opens-up-about-his-in-game-panic-attack/?utm_term=.9917454fc655

Bühlmayer, L., Birrer, D., Röthlin, P., Faude, O., & Donath, L. (2017). Effects of mindfulness practice on performance-relevant parameters and performance outcomes in sports: A meta-analytical review. *Sports Medicine, 47*, 2309–2321. doi:10.1007/s40279-017-0752-9

Clay, R. A. (2017). *A new NFL playbook: Enhancing mental health*. Retrieved from https://www.apa.org/monitor/2017/01/nfl-playbook.aspx

Clement, S., Schauman, O., Graham, T., Maggioni, F., Evans-Lacko, S., Bezborodovs, N., ... Thornicroft, G. (2015). What is the impact of mental health-related stigma on help-seeking? A systematic review of quantitative and qualitative studies. *Psychological Medicine, 45*(1), 11–27. doi:10.1017/S0033291714000129

Cogan, M. (2014, June 25). *The pursuit of "radical acceptance."* Retrieved from http://www.espn.com/nfl/story/_/page/hotread140707/chicago-bears-brandon-marshall-spreads-awareness-nfl-mental-health-crisis-espn-magazine

Constantine, M. G. (1995). Retired female athletes in transition: A group counseling intervention. *Journal of College Student Development, 36*(6), 604–605.

Cunningham, R., & Turner, M. J. (2016). Using rational emotive behavior therapy (REBT) with mixed martial arts (MMA) athletes to reduce irrational beliefs and increase unconditional self-acceptance. *Journal of Rational-Emotive & Cognitive-Behavior Therapy, 34*, 289. doi:10.1007/s10942-016-0240-4

Danish, S. J., Petitpas, A. J., & Hale, B. D. (1993). Life development intervention for athletes: Life skills through sports. *The Counseling Psychologist, 21*(3), 352–385. doi:10.1177/0011000093213002

David, D., Cotet, C., Matu, S., Mogoase, C., & Stefan, S. (2018). 50 years of rational-emotive and cognitive-behavioral therapy: A systematic review and meta-analysis. *Journal of Clinical Psychology, 8*(74), 304–318. doi:10.1002/jclp.22514

Deen, S., Turner, M. J., & Wong, R. S. K. (2017). The effects of REBT, and the use of credos, on irrational beliefs and resilience qualities in athletes. *The Sport Psychologist, 31*(3), 249–263. doi:10.1123/tsp.2016-0057

Didymus, F., & Fletcher, D. (2017). Effects of a cognitive-behavioral intervention on field hockey players' appraisals of organizational stressors. *Psychology of Sport and Exercise, 30.* doi:10.1016/j.psychsport.2017.03.005

Ellis, A. (1957). Rational psychotherapy and individual psychology. *Journal of Individual Psychology, 13*(1), 38.

Gardner, F. L., & Moore, Z. E. (2004). A mindfulness-acceptance-commitment-based approach to athletic performance enhancement: Theoretical considerations. *Behavior Therapy, 35,* 707–723. doi:10.1016/S0005-7894(04)80016-9

Gerrity, D. A., & DeLucia-Waack, J. L. (2006). Effectiveness of groups in the schools. *The Journal for Specialists in Group Work, 32*(1), 97–106. doi:10.1080/01933920600978604

Gleeson, S., & Brady, E. (2017, August 30). *When athletes share their battles with mental illness.* Retrieved from https://www.usatoday.com/story/sports/2017/08/30/michael-phelps-brandon-marshall-mental-health-battles-royce-white-jerry-west/596857001/

Granito, V. J., Hogan, J. B., & Varnum, L. K. (1995). The performance enhancement group program: Integrating sport psychology and rehabilitation. *Journal of Athletic Training, 30*(4), 328–331.

Gross, M., Moore, Z. E., Gardner, F. L., Wolanin, A. T., Pess, R., & Marks, D. R. (2018). An empirical examination comparing the mindfulness-acceptance-commitment approach and psychological skills training for the mental health and sport performance of female student athletes. *International Journal of Sport and Exercise Psychology, 16*(4), 431–451. doi:10.1080/1612197X.2016.1250802

Gustafsson, H. K., & Lundqvist, C. (2016). Working with perfectionism in elite sport: A Cognitive Behavioral Therapy perspective. In Andrew Hill (Ed.), *Perfectionism in sport, dance and exercise* (pp. 203–221). London: Routledge.

Gustafsson, H., Lundqvist, C., & Tod, D. (2017). Cognitive behavioral intervention in sport psychology: A case illustration of the exposure method with an elite athlete. *Journal of Sport Psychology in Action, 8*(3), 152–162. doi:10.1080/21520704.2016.1235649

Harris, H. L., Altekruse, M. K., & Engels, D. W. (2003). Helping freshman student athletes adjust to college life using psychoeducational groups. *The Journal for Specialists in Group Work, 28*(1), 64–81. doi:10.1177/019339202250079

Hays, K. F. (1999). *Working it out: Using exercise in psychotherapy* (pp. 177–187). Washington, DC: American Psychological Association. doi:10.1037/10333-017

Herkov, M. (2016). *What is psychotherapy?* Psych Central. Retrieved from https://psychcentral.com/lib/what-is-psychotherapy/

Hughes, D. (2014, October 10). *Premier League tackling mental health.* Retrieved from https://www.bbc.com/news/health-29543252

Keble, A. (2016, December 5). *Overcoming the empathy barrier: Mental health in the premier league.* Retrieved from https://sports.vice.com/en_uk/article/xybgbn/overcoming-the-empathy-barrier-mental-health-in-the-premier-league

Kliegman, J. (2017, October 26). *College athletes are only starting to get access to the mental health care they need.* Retrieved from https://www.theringer.com/2017/10/26/16535274/ncaa-student-athletes-mental-health-care-initiatives

Linardon, J. (2018). Meta-analysis of the effects of cognitive-behavioral therapy on the core eating disorder maintaining mechanisms: Implications for mechanisms of therapeutic change. *Cognitive Behaviour Therapy*, 47(2), 107–125. doi:10.1080/16506 073.2018.1427785

Mahoney, J., & Hanrahan, S. J. (2011). A brief educational intervention using acceptance and commitment therapy: Four injured athletes' experiences. *Journal of Clinical Sport Psychology*, 5(3), 252–273. doi:10.1123/jcsp.5.3.252

Moreland, J. J., Coxe, K. A, & Yang, J. (2018). Collegiate athletes' mental health services utilization: A systematic review of conceptualizations, operationalizations, facilitators, and barriers. *Journal of Sport and Health Science*, 7(1), 58–69. doi:10.1016/j.jshs.2017.04.009

Mosewich, A. D., Crockdere, P. R. E., Kowalski, K. C., & Delongis, A. (2013). Applying self-compassion in sport: An intervention with women athletes. *Journal of Sport and Exercise Psychology*, 35, 514–524. doi:10.1123/jsep.35.5.514

National Alliance on Mental Illness. (2018). *Psychosocial treatments*. Retrieved from https://www.nami.org/Learn-More/Treatment/Psychosocial-Treatments

Naylor, A., Clement, D., Shannon, V. R., & Cannole, I. J. (2011). Performance enhancement groups for injured athletes. *Athletic Therapy and Training*, 16(3), 34–36. doi:10.1123/ijatt.16.3.34

Noren, N. (2014, January 26). *Taking notice of the hidden injury*. Retrieved from http://www.espn.com/espn/otl/story/_/id/10335925/awareness-better-treatment-college-athletes-mental-health-begins-take-shape

Rapoport, I. (2012, July 26). *"NFL Total Wellness" program launched to improve player health*. Retrieved from http://www.nfl.com/news/story/09000d5d82ad2ab4/printable/nfl-total-wellness-program-launched-to-improve-player-health

Reardon, C.L., & Factor R.M. (2010). Sport psychiatry: A systematic review of diagnosis and medical treatment of mental illness in athletes. Sports Medicine, 40, 961–980. doi:10.2165/11536580-000000000-00000

Reynolds, T. (2018, September 18). *NBA, union reminds players that mental health help available*. Retrieved from http://www.nba.com/article/2018/09/18/nba-union-reminds-players-mental-health-help-available

Saxena, S., Jané-Llopis, E., & Hosman, C. (2006). Prevention of mental and behavioural disorders: Implications for policy and practice. *World Psychiatry: Official Journal of the World Psychiatric Association (WPA)*, 5(1), 5–14.

Splete, H. (2016). Cognitive behavioral therapy eases postconcussive symptoms in teens. *Neurology Reviews*, 24(10), 40.

Steinfeldt, M., & Steinfeldt, J. A. (2012). Athletic identity and conformity to masculine norms among college football players. *Journal of Applied Sport Psychology*, 24(2), 115–128. doi:10.1080/10413200.2011.603405

Stillman, M. A., Brown, T., Ritvo, E. C., & Glick, I. D. (2016). Sport psychiatry and psychotherapeutic intervention, circa 2016. *International Review of Psychiatry*, 28, 614–622. doi:10.1080/09540261.2016.1202812

Turner, M., & Barker, J. B, (2013). Examining the efficacy of rational-emotive behavior therapy (REBT) on irrational beliefs and anxiety in elite youth cricketers. *Journal of Applied Sport Psychology*, 25(1), 131–147. doi:10.1080/10413200.2011.574311

USC Student Health. (n.d.). *Postdoctoral fellowship—Sport psychology*. Retrieved from https://studenthealth.usc.edu/counseling/training-programs/postdoctoral-fellowship-sports/

Vealey, R. S. (2005). *Coaching for the inner edge*. Morgantown, WV: Fitness Information Technology.

Virtual Medical Centre. (2014). *Psychoeducation*. Retrieved from https://www.myvmc.com/treatments/psychoeducation/

Wahto, R. S., Swift, J. K., & Whipple, J. L. (2016). The role of stigma and referral source in predicting college student-athletes' attitudes toward psychological help-seeking. *Journal of Clinical Sport Psychology, 10*(2), 85–98. doi:10.1123/JCSP.2015-0025

Wellander, L., Wells, M. B., & Feldman, I. (2016). Does prevention pay? Costs and potential cost-savings of school interventions targeting children with mental health problems. *The Journal of Mental Health Policy and Economics, 19*, 91–102.

Yalom, I. D. (1995). *The theory and practice of group psychotherapy.* New York, NY: Basic Books.

12

RESILIENCE AND ADVERSARIAL GROWTH

Serena is a high-level golfer with aspirations of playing professionally. A native of Guatemala, she moved to the U.S. a few years prior in search of more opportunities to advance her game. As expected, the transition away from friends and family and into a new country was difficult. Finances have also been a source of stress. Early success in tournaments allowed her to secure some small sponsors, but these have mostly disappeared as she has struggled with her game. Having to work full-time while still devoting the necessary hours to developing her game has been extremely challenging. At the same time, a nagging back injury has hindered her ability to practice and play. Despite all of this, Serena maintained her resolve and a positive attitude. Her friends constantly marveled at her optimism, and the passion she continued to show for golf. Her hard work finally paid off when despite all her struggles, she finished in the top five against a strong field of competitors. When interviewed by a local reporter about her journey, she credited her family for instilling a strong work ethic and providing the opportunity to pursue a career in golf. The discussion turned to the tragic death of her younger brother several years prior, and she explained that although she will always miss him, the experience of working through his passing has strengthened her to handle any obstacle she might face in or out of golf.

Implicit to the discussion of psychosocial "threats," "prevention," and "treatment" is the notion that adverse experiences are necessarily harmful for athletes and should be avoided at all costs. Although the evidence presented in this text confirms the potential for a host of deleterious psychosocial outcomes due to common threats in the sport environment, this does not preclude the possibility that athletes will either: (a) soon return to a pre-threat level of functioning, or (b) emerge from their experience with the threat in some way better off than they were before. Indeed, high-level sport is filled with examples of athletes who have successfully overcome extremely challenging circumstances, and in some cases reported personal benefits because of them. For example, there is the story of U.S. speed skater Dan Jansen, who after falling short of gold medal expectations in three Olympic Games, and enduring the death of his sister shortly before the 1988 Games, broke through in his final race to earn a gold medal in the 1994 Olympics (Giblin, 2018). Or Irish gymnast Kieran Behan, who despite briefly losing the use of his legs at the age of 10 due to complications from a surgery, and then sustaining a serious head injury in training at age 15, went on to become only the second ever Irish Olympic gymnast (Full Twist, 2012). And Muslim American fencer Ibtihaj Muhammed, who overcame a host of racial, gender, and religious biases to become the first American woman to compete in the Olympics while wearing a hijab (Kaplan, 2016).

Whereas the preceding examples illustrate the tendency for high-level athletes to achieve their goals despite obstacles, others have described the transformative impact of their struggles. One case in point is professional basketball player Shaun Livingston, whose career was in serious doubt in 2007 after he suffered a gruesome injury resulting in a dislocated kneecap, sprained medial collateral ligament, torn anterior cruciate ligament, torn posterior cruciate ligament, torn lateral meniscus, and fractured leg (Poole, 2018). He missed an entire season, and then bounced between eight teams over the next six seasons. However, since 2014, he has played a valuable role for the three-time NBA champion Golden State Warriors, and credits his late-career success with the difficulties he experienced beginning with his injury:

> Honestly, it couldn't have worked out any better for me, in terms of my career and the trajectory of everything and how it came about. Being on seven or eight different teams in a matter of six to eight years, it was a lot. A lot of movement. A lot of travel. But it also was a growing experience.
>
> *(Poole, 2018, para. 8)*

In this final chapter I consider the other side of threats to athletes' psychosocial health—resilience and adversarial growth. Both concepts fit conceptually with the notion of psychological well-being, which includes personal growth as one component, and is related to individuals' ability to successfully navigate stressors (Ryff, Love, Essex, & Singer, 1998; Sagone & De Caroli, 2014). First, I consider the concept of resilience, including a summary of its scholarly history outside of sport, and more recent advances within sport. Second, I transition to a similar discussion of adversarial growth. Finally, based on extant research and theory, I offer recommendations for the promotion of resilience and growth in high-level athletes.

Resilience

Long before it was the focus of sport researchers, scholars in the realm of developmental child psychopathology were intrigued by what they observed in longitudinal studies of children born into high-risk conditions (e.g., poverty, parents with psychological illness). Rather than struggle as might be expected, many of the youth developed into well-adjusted and high-functioning young adults (e.g., Rutter, 1985; Werner, 2004). As the scholarly field of resilience expanded, so too did the number of definitions and conceptualizations (see Aburn, Gott, & Hoare, 2016 for a recent review). At the core of the discussion was the extent to which resilience was best measured as a dispositional trait, an outcome, or a dynamic process (Rutter, 2000). Masten, Best, & Garmezy (1990) offered one of the more complete definitions of resilience when they stated that it refers to "the process of, capacity for, or outcome of successful adaptation despite challenging or threatening circumstances" (p. 425). Central to this and other definitions of resilience are three criteria: (a) adversity (e.g., poverty, acute trauma) (b) factors buffering individuals from long-term difficulties due to the adversity (e.g., personal and environmental factors), and (c) successful adaptation despite the adversity (e.g., lack of psychological disorder, degree of psychological adjustment).

As data accumulated in support of seemingly "rare" instances of positive adaptation to chronic stress, Masten (2001) coined the term *ordinary magic* to characterize how the capacity of individuals to successfully adapt to stressful circumstances, although remarkable, results from the presence of personal and environmental factors that are actually quite common. Indeed, resilience is the most typical response among adults who have experienced acute trauma (Bonanno, 2004). Research since the 1980's has revealed several personal and environmental factors related to positive outcomes despite the presence of high-risk situations for youth (Werner, 2000). Personal protective factors for resilience include strong emotion regulation, social competence, positive self-concept, and an internal locus of control (Dahlin & Cederblad, 1993; Werner, 2000). Common environmental protective factors include the presence of caring relationships, positive role models, high expectations, and opportunities for leadership (Werner, 1995). Subsequent research has resulted in lists of protective factors and their link to positive outcomes in specific sub-groups of children and adults (e.g., Bonanno, 2004; Hamby, Grych, & Banyard, 2018; Jocson, Alers-Rojas, Ceballo, & Arkin, 2018; Schaefer, Howell, Schwartz, Bottomley, & Crossnine, 2018).

Because high-level sport is by nature filled with challenges and obstacles for participants, it is a natural context from which to examine resilience. Despite recent advancements, the study of sport resilience continues to be plagued by a lack of consistency in the conceptualization, operationalization, and measurement of the construct (Galli & Gonzalez, 2015; Sarkar & Fletcher, 2013). Nonetheless, a handful of studies have made useful contributions to researchers' understanding of the protective factors and positive outcomes experienced by high-level sport performers. In the remainder of this section I highlight the results of sport resilience studies most relevant to this text, which include those focused on high-level athletes who have adapted well cognitively, emotionally, socially, and/or spiritually to threats/adversities in the sport environment. Further, because of inconsistencies in measurement, and problems associated with labeling individuals as "resilient" vs. "non-resilient" noted by Luthar and Cicchetti (2000), I emphasize studies operationalizing resilience as an outcome or process rather than a self-reported aspect of personality.

Much of the research on resilience in high-level athletes conducted in the past decade has focused on protective factors most relevant for promoting positive outcomes despite threats in the sport environment. Researchers studying injury, organizational stress, and burnout in sport have found support for several factors, including social support, coping skills, and positive coach behaviors (Smith, Smoll, & Ptacek, 1990; White & Bennie, 2015). In their comprehensive review, Sarkar and Fletcher (2014) identified additional protective factors from the literature, including positive personality (e.g., adaptive perfectionism, optimism, competitiveness), motivation, confidence, and focus. As compared to earlier research with high-risk youth, socio-environmental protective factors are notably less prominent. Although this may be due to the difference in adversities/threats and outcomes of interest between the groups, it could also be due to the pre-conceived notions of resilience by sport researchers as a personal ability rather than one arising from a mixture of personal and environmental factors. Fortunately, researchers have begun considering the role of important others in the sport environment, such as coaches, in the promotion of resilience in athletes (e.g., Kegelaers & Wylleman, 2018).

Several of the protective factors discussed in Sarkar and Fletcher's (2014) review arose from two qualitative studies of resilience in high-level athletes. Both studies also shed light on psychosocial outcomes resulting from protective factors. The first of these studies was by Galli and Vealey (2008), who interviewed ten current and former high-level athletes regarding the most difficult adversity that they ever experienced in their athletic career (e.g., injury, transition). The authors analyzed the results both deductively according to Richardson et al.'s (Richardson, Neiger, Jensen, & Kumpfer's, 1990) Resiliency Model, and inductively based on athletes' perceptions of their experience. The results informed the development of a conceptual model of sport resilience, in which sport adversities faced by the athletes resulted in a process of agitation characterized by unpleasant emotions and mental struggles, mixed with cognitive and behavioral coping strategies. This process influenced positive outcomes such as increased learning, increased motivation to help others, and a broadened life perspective. However, positive outcomes were also a product of pre-existing sociocultural (e.g., social support) and personal (e.g., achievement motivation) resources. The Galli and Vealey (2008) model has since been adopted and supported in studies of athletes with acquired disabilities (Machida, Irwin, & Feltz, 2013) and survivors of the 2014 Boston Marathon bombings (Timm, Kamphoff, Galli, & Gonzalez, 2017).

Thus, similar to high-risk youth, when athletes possess adequate personal and environmental protective factors they are able to successfully navigate many of the threats to psychosocial health discussed in this text. Furthermore, and as I delineate later in this chapter, the process of negotiating threats may bolster pre-existing protective factors, or even foster the development of new resources to handle future threats.

The second qualitative study of resilience in high-level sport was by Fletcher and Sarkar (2012), who undertook a grounded theory study of psychological resilience in 12 former Olympic champions. In the theory that emerged, psychological resilience was conceptualized as an overarching concept which framed the athletes' responses to sport stressors. Multiple psychological factors, including having a positive personality, motivation, focus, confidence, and perceived social support, influenced performers to appraise stressors as challenges rather than problems, and evaluate their own thinking (i.e., meta-cognition). Challenge appraisals and meta-cognition led to facilitative responses such as increased task engagement, which then led to optimal sport performance. As Fletcher and Sarkar (2012) acknowledged, one weakness of this study is that participants won their gold medal as much as 40 years prior to their interview, making recall bias of greater concern in this study. Further, as mentioned previously, the proposed model offers little reference to the influence of socio-environmental factors on athletes' ability to positively adapt, which have been suggested as important in other qualitative studies of resilience in sport (e.g., Galli & Vealey, 2008; Machida, Irwin, & Feltz, 2013), as well as by scholars who advocate for a process-view of resilience (e.g., Vanderbilt-Adriance & Shaw, 2008; Windle, 2011). Despite its limitations, the Fletcher and Sarkar study was an important step for resilience research in sport, as it introduced meta-cognition as a viable part of resilience for athletes, and offered the first context-specific definition of resilience in sport- "the role of mental processes and behavior in promoting personal assets and protecting an individual from the potential negative effect of stressors" (Fletcher & Sarkar, 2012, p. 675).

Adversarial growth

It is commonplace for athletes, coaches, and others in the high-level sport environment to refer to resilient athletes as those who not only adapt successfully to threats in the sport environment but emerge better than they were before. As Friedrich Nietzsche famously suggested, that which does not kill us only makes us stronger (Nietzsche, 1889). A modern description of Nietzsche's insight was offered by several researchers in the 1990's, who began exploring the potential for positive personal outcomes due to stress and trauma (Park, Cohen, & Murch, 1996; Tedeschi & Calhoun, 1996). And although both resilience and growth represent adaptive responses to adversity, they are not the same. Whereas the resilience trajectory is characterized by a brief period of minimal distress followed by a return to baseline psychosocial functioning, adversarial growth implies psychosocial enhancement due to individuals' experience with adversity (Bonanno & Diminich, 2013; Westphal & Bonanno, 2007). As Westphal and Bonanno (2007) argued, people who are resilient have little need or opportunity to grow from adversity. I now provide a brief overview of theories and models of adversarial growth (aka posttraumatic growth, stress-related growth), followed by a review of the literature on adversarial growth in high-level athletes.

Two theories have been particularly influential in explaining how individuals might be improved by adversity. The functional-descriptive model proposed by Tedeschi and Calhoun (1995) posits that the process of growth is triggered by "seismic event" which challenges individuals' fundamental beliefs about the world. As individuals experience automatic and intrusive thoughts (i.e., ruminate) about the issue, they begin to self-disclose through by talking to others, writing, and praying. Self-disclosure promotes a sense of social support, which in turn leads to reduced distress, and more intentional cognitive processing characterized by the formation of new narratives about their adverse experience and life in general. It is because of this more deliberate ruminative activity that growth occurs in one or more areas. Specifically, based on extant literature and their own clinical practice, Tedeschi and Calhoun (1996) suggested five domains of growth: (a) increased appreciation for life (e.g., "I am more grateful for the little things"), (b) closer relationships with others (e.g., "I now know who my real friends are"), (c) increased personal strength (e.g., "I know now that I can handle more than I believed"), (d) identification of new possibilities (e.g., "Because of what my physical therapist did for me, I want to do the same for others"), and (e) spiritual growth (e.g., "I have a stronger faith in God"). An important element of the functional-descriptive model is the recognition that growth does not necessarily preclude distress. In fact, Calhoun and Tedeschi suggest that some level of enduring distress may even be necessary for sustained growth.

A second theory of adversarial growth was proposed by Joseph and Linley (2005), who drew from positive psychology to propose their organismic-valuing theory of growth (OVT). Like Calhoun and Tedeschi's (1995) assertion that the process of growth is set off by a "seismic event," in OVT growth can only occur when an event is significant enough to shatter individuals' assumptions about the world. Individuals are then driven to integrate new information with their pre-existing understanding of the world, which happens through a mix of cognitive and emotional processing. The extent to which individuals' social environment satisfies their needs for competence, autonomy, and relatedness will determine whether they experience growth. In support of Calhoun and Tedeschi (1995), Joseph and Linley noted that whereas individuals who experience growth may emerge wiser and more appreciative (i.e., eudaimonia), it is not essential that individuals experience positive emotions such as joy or happiness (i.e., subjective well-being). I now highlight several such investigations of adversarial growth in high-level sport.

Although growth was noted as an outcome in a study of season-ending injuries in skiers (Udry, Gould, Bridges, & Beck, 1997) and the aforementioned investigation of resilience (Galli & Vealey, 2008), Galli and Reel (2012) were the first to systematically explore the phenomenon in high-level athletes. Interviews with 11 collegiate athletes who reported at least a moderate degree of growth due to their most difficult sport stressor in the past six months, as measured by Tedeschi and Calhoun's (1996) Posttraumatic Growth Inventory, informed the development of a conceptual model of adversarial growth in athletes. The model illustrates the process of growth reported by participants, in which a combination of struggling to work through their stressor and social support were instrumental in facilitating personal growth in the form of a new life philosophy, self-changes, and interpersonal changes. Athletes' sociocultural context (e.g., family dynamics, race/ethnicity) and personality characteristics (e.g., passion, achievement motivation) both framed and shaped the process. The results support several aspects of Tedeschi and Calhoun's (1995) functional-descriptive model, including the important roles of social support and cognitive processing, as well as the domains of growth.

Since the initial investigation by Galli and Reel (2012), researchers have examined growth in Paralympic athletes (Day, 2013), female athletes (Neely, Dunn, McHugh, & Holt, 2018; Tamminena, Holt, & Neely, 2013), and Olympic swimming champions (Howells & Fletcher, 2015). A consistent finding across studies is the importance of meaning-making and social support in setting the stage for adversarial growth. Unique to Day's (2013) study was the importance of physical activity in laying the foundation for growth in Paralympians who had acquired a traumatic disability. Specifically, the athletes noted how sport allowed them to acknowledge both their limitations and their possibilities, and the ability to take risks and accept responsibility for their actions.

Howells and Fletcher's (2015) study of adversarial growth was unique in that they analyzed content from the autobiographies of Olympic swimming champions. As interpreted by Howells and Fletcher, the story arc of the swimmers tended to show a pattern of initial adversity (e.g., congenital impairments such as dyslexia, abuse, depression), followed by a process of transition characterized by an attempt to maintain a sense of normality through swimming, questioning the win-at-all-costs culture of elite sport, a search for meaning, and social support. The transition ultimately allowed swimmers to experience growth in several realms, including performance, relationships, and spirituality. The long-term narrative accounts of adversity and high-level sport participation offered by swimmers' autobiographies allowed the researchers to obtain a "landscape" view of the growth process not usually available in traditional research designs.

The most developed line of research devoted to adversarial growth in sport is led by Wadey et al. (e.g., Salim, Wadey, & Diss, 2016; Wadey, Evans, Evans, & Mitchell, 2011), who have conducted a series of quantitative and qualitative investigations to understand the process and outcomes of growth in injured athletes (i.e., sport injury-related growth; Roy-Davis, Wadey, & Evans, 2018. In his initial study, Wadey et al. (2011) analyzed interviews with ten high-level athletes to understand the antecedents, mechanisms, and growth outcomes in each phase of injury recovery. For example, growth due to injury onset was spurred by emotional responses, prompting athletes to self-disclose and seek support from others, and resulting in an enhanced ability to understand, express, and regulate emotions. One intriguing finding was athletes' perception of enhanced resilience as an outcome of the return to sport process, suggesting a link between the two constructs that awaits further investigation. Wadey et al. quantitatively identified pathways to growth, such as the mediational effect of emotional support seeking and positive reframing on the relationship between hardiness and growth (Salim et al., 2016). Wadey, Podlog, Galli, and Mellalieu (2016) found preliminary support for the OVT as an explanation for growth due to sport injury, as growth mediated the relationship between need satisfaction (i.e., competence and relatedness) and subjective well-being.

Roy-Davis, Wadey, and Evans (2018) recently conducted the most in-depth investigation of sport-injury growth to date. After an impressive 70 interviews with 37 athletes conducted over 24 months, the researchers developed a comprehensive grounded theory of sport-injury related growth (SIRG). Many of the components of the theory supported extant research on resilience and growth, including the important roles played by positive personality, meta-cognition, previous experiences with adversity, social support, and effective coping in facilitating growth. Further, the various domains of growth (e.g., increased personal strength, enhanced social relationships, increased pro-social behavior) noted by athletes aligned with previous studies of adversarial growth in sport. Novel findings included the influence of *cultural scripts,* or narratives of triumphing over adversity portrayed in the media, as inspiring participants to do the same. Most importantly, the grounded theory of SIRG represents the most complete sport-specific theory of adversarial growth to date, and an ideal starting point for future research in the area.

Promoting resilience and growth in high-level athletes

Given the threats to psychosocial health inherent to the high-level sport environment presented in Chapters 4–8, the promotion of resilience and adversarial growth should be a high priority for sport leaders. Research and theory from within and outside of sport offer insight for how athletes can bounce back from such threats, and perhaps realize growth because of them. Two frameworks, one from the study of high-risk children, and another specific to performers, are particularly informative for promoting resilience in high-level athletes.

Benard's (1997) resiliency framework provides guidelines for creating an environment in which individuals' innate capacity for resilience is activated. Within the framework, three envirosocial protective factors are highlighted: (a) caring relationships, (b) high expectations, and (c) opportunities for participation and contribution. The three factors are interactive, such that the presence of each maximizes the benefit of the others. Individuals exposed to environments supportive of these conditions are more likely to display social competence, a strong sense of identity, problem-solving, and optimism (Benard, 1991). Although Benard's framework was not designed with the high-level sport environment in mind, it is easy to envision how a collegiate, Olympic, or professional coach might consider these three protective factors for building a resilient team. She might work to create a team setting wherein athletes trust and respect one another and feel safe discussing concerns with the coaching staff (i.e., caring relationships). The presence of caring relationships would provide the foundation for the coach to rely on athlete strengths for goal achievement and athletes sense a belief from their coach that they have the capacity to meet her high expectations. Once athletes feel cared for and understand the coach's expectations for their effort and attitude, she would ideally provide frequent opportunities for them to live up to these expectations in practice and games. An important aspect of such opportunities is the opportunity to fall short of expectations and learn from those disappointments. When the three conditions of caring relationships, high expectations, and opportunities are consistently present, athletes will be better equipped to tap into their innate capacity for resilience when handling the sport-specific threats discussed in this text.

A second framework for fostering resilience is Fletcher and Sarkar's (2016) mental fortitude training model. Based on research on stress and resilience in sport, Fletcher and Sarkar identify three essential factors for promoting resilience in high-level athletes: (a) personal qualities, (b) a facilitative environment, and (c) a challenge mindset. In brief, the authors posit that athletes' internal protective factors (e.g., personality traits and psychological skills) are maximized when training and competing in an environment which balances support with challenge. The byproduct of the bidirectional relationship between personal qualities and a facilitative environment is a challenge mindset, characterized by functional appraisals of sport-specific threats by athletes. Athletes are more likely to positively adapt to threats when they view them as opportunities, and recognize the unique personal qualities that can help them to succeed despite adversity.

Thus, like Benard's (1997) framework, Fletcher and Sarkar highlight the environment as critical for the expression of personal protective factors in the presence of sport threats. And while it is likely that in-born personality traits cause some athletes to have a wider "resilience bandwidth" than others (Fletcher & Sarkar, 2016), sport leaders can ensure that athletes reach their resilience potential by teaching athletes psychological skills such as attentional focus and emotion regulation and allowing opportunity to practice these skills within challenging yet supportive sport environments. Although Fletcher and Sarkar's model seems most applicable to performance-specific threats (i.e., performance pressure) rather than threats further removed from the performance setting (e.g., abuse, transition), as the only sport-specific resilience training program, it warrants consideration from researchers and practitioners broadly interested in building athlete resilience. Randomized controlled trials will allow for an understanding of the effectiveness of the program for promoting positive psychosocial as well as performance outcomes in response to a variety of the threats discussed in this text.

In terms of proactively setting the conditions for adversarial growth in sport, we can learn from extant research and theory. According to the OVT, environmental conditions that meet individuals' needs for competence, autonomy, and relatedness provide the energy for growth. Wadey et al.'s (2016) study of growth due to sport injury partially supported the OVT, as athletes' perceptions of competence and relatedness were linked to growth, which in turn predicted subjective well-being. Thus, at least as it relates to injury, sport leaders should work to promote a sense of proficiency as athletes recover, highlighting the attainment of milestones and improvements along the way. Further, keeping injured athletes involved with the team at some level would enhance perceptions of relatedness, which offers a second potential pathway for growth.

The issue of promoting adversarial growth after difficult events have occurred is somewhat controversial. In the non-sport literature, clinicians caution against *expecting* that clients achieve growth through their struggles, and instead be vigilant about listening for signs that they are recognizing potential enhancements themselves (Calhoun & Tedeschi, 2012). As suggested by the functional descriptive model of growth, the process of growth partially stems from the kind of social support and opportunity for cognitive processing often provided by psychotherapy. Although not all athletes will require or use psychotherapy, emotional disclosure of thoughts and feelings about their struggles remains a viable avenue for growth. Indeed, Salim and Wadey (2018) found that previously injured athletes who engaged in four 20-minute sessions of verbal disclosure about their injury into an audio recorder reported significantly more adversarial growth than participants in a control or written disclosure group. Despite this finding, the authors noted the challenge faced by sport organizations to de-stigmatize efforts by athletes to talk about their struggles, problems, and concerns. That is, the narrative around emotional disclosure should be changed from one of weakness to one of empowerment for growth. By providing physical space and trained support staff to facilitate emotional disclosure, sport organizations would send a message to athletes that it is ok, and even encouraged, to verbalize their personal struggles (Salim & Wadey, 2018).

Conclusion

In this chapter I recognized the potential for athletes to successfully adapt to and grow from threats in the sport environment. After first drawing from research with non-sport populations, studies with high-level athletes in the last decade has led researchers to develop sport-specific models and theories of resilience and adversarial growth. Both general and sport theories serve as a blueprint for the creation of sport environments conducive to resilience and growth in the face of threats to athletes' psychosocial health and well-being. The next step for researchers is to go beyond descriptive studies to test the efficacy of resilience and growth interventions. An additional challenge for researchers is to ascertain which elements of the resilience and growth processes are universal to all sport-specific threats, and which are unique to specific threats. An understanding of these nuances will allow for the development of selective programming based on the needs of certain athletes rather than a one-size-fits-all approach. Despite the many threats to psychosocial health posed by high-level sport, it is also fertile ground for the promotion of factors which allow athletes to successfully thrive despite adversity on and off the field of play.

References

Aburn, G., Gott, M., & Hoare, K. (2016). What is resilience? An integrative review of the empirical literature. *Journal of Advanced Nursing, 72*, 980–1000. doi:10.1111/jan.12888

Benard, G. (1991, August). *Fostering resiliency in kids: Protective factors in the family, school, and community.* ERIC/CUE Digest. Retrieved from https://eric.ed.gov/?id=ed335781

Benard, B. (1997, August). *Turning it around for all youth: From risk to resilience.* ERIC/CUE Digest, Number 126. Retrieved from https://eric.ed.gov/?id=ED412309

Bonanno, G. A. (2004). Loss, trauma, and human resilience: Have we underestimated the human capacity to thrive after extremely aversive events? *American Psychologist, 59*(1), 20–28. doi:10.1037/0003-066X.59.1.20

Bonanno, G. A., & Diminich, E. D. (2013). Annual research review: Positive adjustment to adversity—trajectories of minimal-impact resilience and emergent resilience. *Journal of Child Psychology and Psychiatry, 54*, 378–401. doi:10.1111/jcpp.12021

Calhoun, L. G., & Tedeschi, R. G. (2012). *Posttraumatic growth in clinical practice.* New York, NY: Routledge.

Dahlin, L., & Cederblad, M. (1993). Salutogenesis-protective factors for individuals brought up in a high-risk environment with regard to the risk for a psychiatric or social disorder. *Nordic Journal of Psychiatry, 47*, 53–60.

Day, M. C. (2013). The role of initial physical activity experiences in promoting posttraumatic growth in Paralympic athletes with an acquired disability. *Disability and Rehabilitation, 35*, 2064–2072. doi:10.3109/09638288.2013.805822

Fletcher, D., & Sarkar, M. (2012). A grounded theory of psychological resilience in Olympic champions. *Psychology of Sport and Exercise, 13*, 669–678. doi:10.1016/j.psychsport.2012.04.007

Fletcher, D., & Sarkar, M. (2016). Mental fortitude training: An evidence-based approach to developing psychological resilience for sustained success. *Journal of Sport Psychology in Action, 7*(3), 135–157. doi:10.1080/21520704.2016.1255496

Full Twist. (2012, January 10). *Kieran Behan—Preparing for London.* Retrieved from http://fulltwist.net/9401/

Galli, N., & Gonzalez, S. P. (2015). Psychological resilience in sport: A review of the literature and implications for research and practice. *International Journal of Sport and Exercise Psychology, 13*(3), 243–257. doi:10.1080/1612197X.2014.946947

Galli, N., & Reel, J. J. (2012). "It was hard, but it was good": A qualitative exploration of stress-related growth in Division I intercollegiate athletes. *Qualitative Research in Sport, Exercise and Health, 4*(3), 297–319. doi:10.1080/2159676X.2012.693524

Galli, N., & Vealey, R. S. (2008). "Bouncing back" from adversity: Athletes' experiences of resilience. *The Sport Psychologist, 22*(3), 316–335. doi:10.1123/tsp.22.3.316

Giblin, C. (2018). *The 10 most unforgettable moments in Winter Olympics history.* Retrieved from https://www.mensjournal.com/sports/the-10-most-unforgettable-moments-in-olympic-history/6-1994-dan-jansen-finally-takes-the-gold/

Hamby, S., Grych, J., & Banyard, V. (2018). Resilience portfolios and poly-strengths: Identifying protective factors associated with thriving after adversity. *Psychology of Violence, 8*(2), 172–183. doi:10.1037/vio0000135

Howells, K., & Fletcher, D. (2015). Sink or swim: Adversity- and growth-related experiences in Olympic swimming champions. *Psychology of Sport and Exercise, 16*(3), 37–48. doi:10.1016/j.psychsport.2014.08.004

Jocson, R. M., Alers-Rojas, F., Ceballo, R., & Arkin, M. (2018). Religion and spirituality: Benefits for Latino adolescents exposed to community violence. *Youth & Society.* doi:10.1177/0044118X18772714

Joseph, S., & Linley, P. A. (2005). Positive adjustment to threatening events: An organismic valuing theory of growth through adversity. *Review of General Psychology, 9*(3), 262–280. doi.:10.1037/1089-2680.9.3.262

Kaplan, S. (2016, March 14). *Meet Ibtihaj Muhammad, the history-making Olympian who called out SXSW for telling her to remove her hijab.* Retrieved from https://www.washingtonpost.com/news/morning-mix/wp/2016/03/14/meet-ibtihaj-muhammad-the-history-making-olympian-who-called-out-sxsw-for-telling-her-to-remove-her-hijab/?utm_term=.931c638c8a9c

Kegelaers, J., Wylleman, P., De Brandt, K., Van Rossem, N., & Rosier, N. (2018). Incentives and deterrents for drug-taking behaviour in elite sports: A holistic and developmental approach. *European Sport Management Quarterly, 18*(1), 112–132. doi:10.1080/16184742.2017.1384505

Luthar, S., & Cicchetti, D. (2000). The construct of resilience: Implications for interventions and social policies. *Development and Psychopathology, 12*(4), 857–885.

Machida, M., Irwin, B., & Feltz, D. (2013). Resilience in competitive athletes with spinal cord injury: The role of sport participation. *Qualitative Health Research, 23,* 1054–1065. doi:10.1177/1049732313493673

Masten, A., Best, K., & Garmezy, N. (1990). Resilience and development: Contributions from the study of children who overcome adversity. *Development and Psychopathology, 2*(4), 425–444. doi:10.1017/S0954579400005812

Masten, A. S. (2001). Ordinary magic: Resilience processes in development. *American Psychologist, 56*(3), 227–238.

Neely, K. C., Dunn, J. G. H., McHugh, T.-L. F., & Holt, N. L. (2018). Female athletes' experiences of positive growth following deselection in sport. *Journal of Sport & Exercise Psychology, 40*(4), 173–185. doi:10.1123/jsep.2017-0136

Nietzsche, F. (2009). *Twilight of the idols: Or how to philosophize with a hammer* (D. Large, Trans.). Oxford, United Kingdom: Oxford University Press.

Park, C. L., Cohen, L. H., & Murch, R. L. (1996). Assessment and prediction of stress-related growth. *Journal of Personality, 64,* 71–105. doi:10.1111/j.1467-6494.1996.tb00815.x

Poole, M. (2018, October 3). *Shaun Livingston living in the moment, shrugs off hazy Warriors future.* Retrieved from https://www.nbcsports.com/bayarea/warriors/shaun-livingston-living-moment-shrugs-hazy-warriors-future

Richardson, G. E., Neiger, B. L., Jensen, S., & Kumpfer, K. L. (1990). The Resiliency Model. *Health Education, 21*(6), 33–39. doi:10.1080/00970050.1990.10614589

Roy-Davis, K., Wadey, R., & Evans, L. (2017). A grounded theory of sport injury-related growth. *Sport, Exercise, and Performance Psychology, 6*(1), 35–52. Retrieved from http://dx.doi.org/10.1037/spy0000080

Rutter, M. (1985). Resilience in the face of adversity: Protective factors and resistance to psychiatric disorder. *British Journal of Psychiatry, 147,* 598–691. doi:10.1192/bjp.147.6.598

Rutter, M. (2000). Resilience reconsidered: Conceptual considerations, empirical findings, and policy implications. In J. P. Shonkoff & S. J. Meisels (Eds.), *Handbook of early childhood intervention* (pp. 651–682). New York, NY: Cambridge University Press. doi:10.1017/CBO9780511529320.030

Ryff, C. D., Singer, B., Love, G. D., & Essex, M. J. (1998). Resilience in adulthood and later life: Defining features and dynamic processes. In J. Lomranz (Ed.), *Handbook of aging and mental health: An integrative approach* (pp. 69–96). New York, NY: Plenum Press.

Sagone, E., & De Caroli, M. E. (2014). Relationships between psychological well-being and resilience in middle and late adolescents. *Procedia—Social and Behavioral Sciences, 141*, 881–887.

Salim, J., & Wadey, R. (2018). Can emotional disclosure promote sport injury-related growth? *Journal of Applied Sport Psychology, 30*(4), 367–387. doi:10.1080/10413200.2017.1417338

Salim, J., Wadey, R., & Diss, C. (2016). Examining hardiness, coping and stress-related growth following sport injury. *Journal of Applied Sport Psychology, 28*(2), 154–169. doi:10.1080/10413200.2015.1086448

Sarkar, M., & Fletcher, D. (2013). How should we measure psychological resilience in sport performers? *Measurement in Physical Education and Exercise Science, 17*(4), 264–280. doi:10.1080/1091367X.2013.805141

Sarkar, M., & Fletcher, D. (2014). Psychological resilience in sport performers: A review of stressors and protective factors. *Journal of Sports Sciences, 32*, 1419–1434. doi:10.1080/02640414.2014.901551

Schaefer, L. M., Howell, K. H., Schwartz, L. E., Bottomley, J. S., & Crossnine, C. B. (2018). A concurrent examination of protective factors associated with resilience and posttraumatic growth following childhood victimization. *Child Abuse & Neglect, 85*, 17–27. doi:10.1016/j.chiabu.2018.08.019

Smith, R. E., Smoll, F. L., & Ptacek, J. T. (1990). Conjunctive moderator variables in vulnerability and resiliency research: Life stress, social support and coping skills, and adolescent sport injuries. *Journal of Personality and Social Psychology, 58*(2), 360–370.

Tamminena, K. A., Holt, N. L., & Neely, K. C. (2013). Exploring adversity and the potential for growth among elite female athletes. *Psychology of Sport and Exercise, 14*(1), 28–36. doi:10.1016/j.psychsport.2012.07.002

Tedeschi, R. G., & Calhoun, L. G. (1995). *Trauma & transformation: Growing in the aftermath of suffering.* Thousand Oaks, CA: SAGE.

Tedeschi, R. G., & Calhoun, L. G. (1996). The Posttraumatic Growth Inventory: Measuring the positive legacy of trauma. *Journal of Traumatic Stress, 9*, 455–471. doi:10.1007/BF02103658

Timm, K., Kamphoff, C., Galli, N., & Gonzalez, S. P. (2017). Resilience and growth in marathon runners in the aftermath of the 2013 Boston Marathon bombings. *The Sport Psychologist, 3*(1), 42–55. doi:10.1123/tsp.2015-0053

Udry, E., Gould, D., Bridges, D., & Beck, L. (1997). Down but not out: Athlete responses to season-ending injuries. *Journal of Sport & Exercise Psychology, 19*(3), 229–248.

Vanderbilt-Adriance, E., & Shaw, D. S. (2008). Conceptualizing and re-evaluating resilience across levels of risk, time, and domains of competence. *Clinical Child and Family Psychology Review, 11*, 30. doi:10.1007/s10567-008-0031-2

Wadey, R., Evans, L., Evans, K., & Mitchell, I. (2011). Perceived benefits following sport injury: A qualitative examination of their antecedents and underlying mechanisms. *Journal of Applied Sport Psychology, 23*(2), 142–158. doi:10.1080/10413200.2010.543119

Wadey, R., Podlog, L., Galli, N., & Mellalieu, S. D. (2016). Organismic valuing theory. *Scandinavian Journal of Medicine & Science in Sports, 26*, 1132–1139. doi:10.1111/sms.12579

Werner, E. E. (1995). Resilience in development. *Current Directions in Psychological Science, 4*(3), 81–84. doi:10.1111/1467-8721.ep10772327

Werner, E. E. (2000). Protective factors and individual resilience. In J. P. Shonkoff & S. J. Meisels (Eds.), Handbook of early intervention (2nd ed., pp. 115–132). New York, NY: Cambridge University Press.

Werner, E. E. (2004). Journeys from childhood to midlife: Risk, resilience, and recovery. *Pediatrics, 114*(2). doi:10.1542/peds.114.2.492

Westphal, M., & Bonanno, G. A. (2007). Posttraumatic growth and resilience to trauma: Different sides of the same coin or different coins? *Applied Psychology, 56*, 417–427. doi:10.1111/j.1464-0597.2007.00298.x

White, R. L., & Bennie, A. (2015). Resilience in youth sport: A qualitative investigation of gymnastics coach and athlete perceptions. *International Journal of Sports Science & Coaching, 10*(2–3), 379–393. doi:10.1260/1747-9541.10.2-3.379

Windle, G. (2011). What is resilience? A review and concept analysis. *Reviews in Clinical Gerontology, 21*(2), 152–169. doi:10.1017/S0959259810000420

INDEX

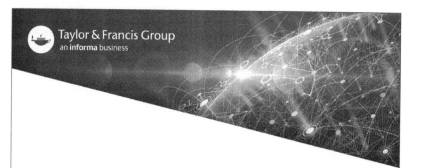